Facial Cupping
MASTERY

Morgan Sutherland, L.M.T.

Facial Cupping Mastery

Copyright © 2019 Morgan Sutherland, L.M.T.

All rights reserved.

No part of this book may be reproduced in any form without permission in writing from the author. Reviewers may quote brief passages in reviews. The information contained in this book is current at the time of this writing. Although all attempts have been made to verify the information provided in this publication, neither the author nor the publisher assume any responsibility for errors, omissions, or contrary interpretations of the subject matter herein.

This book is for educational purposes only. The views expressed are those of the author alone and should not be taken as expert instruction or commands. The reader is responsible for his or her own actions.

At times links might be used to illustrate a point, technique, or best practice. These will reference products I have found useful, but please do your own research, make appropriate comparisons, and form your own decisions as to which products will work best for you. Links to products are used to illustrate points, because they are the examples with which I am most familiar.

Photos: Copyright Morgan Sutherland

Illustrations: Online images, labeled for reuse

Cover image: Copyright Morgan Sutherland

Contents

Facial Cupping

Cupping has been around for thousands of years. Only in the past 10 to 15 years has it become quite the buzzword. Countless celebrities and athletes have posted cupping selfies on social media showing their freshly made circles.

Cupping works great on the back, shoulders, hips, and legs for loosening tight, overworked muscles. But did you know that it also works great on the face? Some even say that it's like Photoshopping a face.

Facial cupping is great for:

- increasing local circulation of the skin;

- helping to reduce facial edema, chronic puffiness, and sinus problems;

- helping to plump and soften expression lines, wrinkles, and scar tissue; and

- reducing tightness and tension in facial muscles associated with temporomandibular (TMJ) dysfunction.

Protocols for the face use small-size glass cups to vacuum and lift the facial tissue, mimicking the pumping movements of lymphatic drainage. It's painless and quite sedating, and several of my clients have drifted off and begun to snore. Others have giggled at the suctioning sound, which resembles little fish kissing their cheeks.

Cupping Massage
M A S T E R Y

Contraindications for Facial Cupping

- Never glide across the carotid or jugular region.

- Do not combine facial cupping with aggressive exfoliation.

- Do not cup open wounds or areas of inflammation on the face.

- Post cupping, clients should avoid exposure to cold/windy weather, hot showers, baths, saunas, hot tubs, and aggressive exercise for at least six hours. Such exposure can produce undesirable effects.

- Post cupping, clients should avoid wearing makeup for six hours to allow the subcutaneous skin layer to reap the benefits of the treatment.

- If clients have had Botox on their face, tread lightly, so as not to do more harm. I've heard some say to wait six months before treating.

Recommended Glass Facial Cupping Set

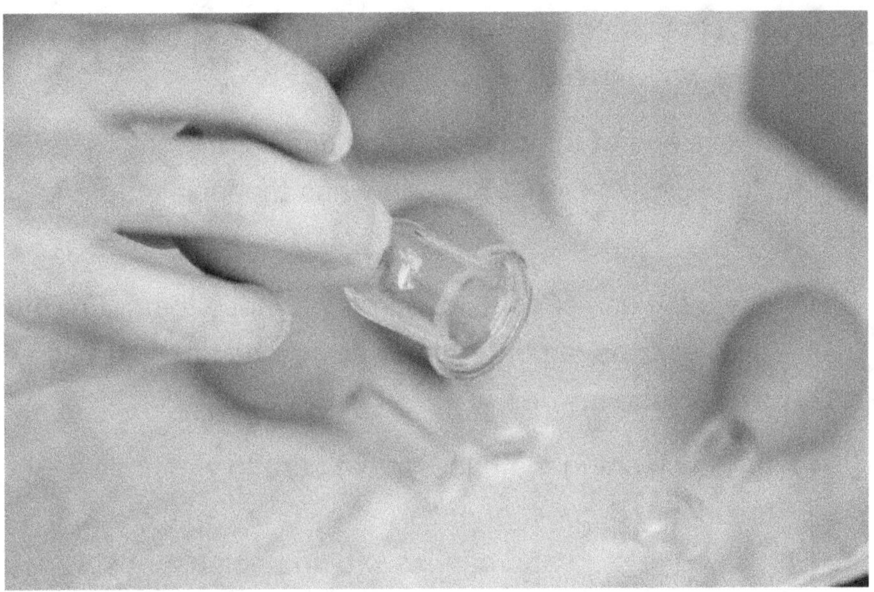

Go to **CuppingMassageMastery.com/resources** to see my recommended facial cupping set.

Caring for Your Facial Cupping Set

After use, clean the cups with a 60:40 ratio of original Listerine to water in a spray bottle.

- At the end of the day, you can use Dr. Bronner's Pure-Castile Liquid Soap to wash the facial cupping set.

- Dry the glass cups as soon as you rinse them. For the smaller cups, a cotton-tip swab can be helpful to wipe and dry the insides.

- When cleaning the cups, make sure to wash the bulbs, but do not squeeze them. This can get water inside the bulb and can lead to an unpleasant surprise for the client during a facial cupping session.

Cupping Massage Mastery
(Video Course)

Take your cupping skills to the next level with the Cupping Massage video training.

In this video course, you'll learn step-by-step treatments for various common chronic pain conditions using user-friendly and flexible silicone cups.

Go to CuppingMassageMastery.com to learn more.

I look forward to seeing you inside the course.

In good health,

Morgan Sutherland, L.M.T.

Instructor, Cupping Massage Mastery

CuppingMassageMastery.com

Facial Cupping Sequence

Total time: 30 minutes.

Begin with the client in the supine position with the therapist seated at the head of the table.

Place the four facial cups you plan to use on the same side of the face you will be working. The photo below shows me placing the cups to the right side of the client's head, because I'm going to begin the facial cupping session on the right side of her face.

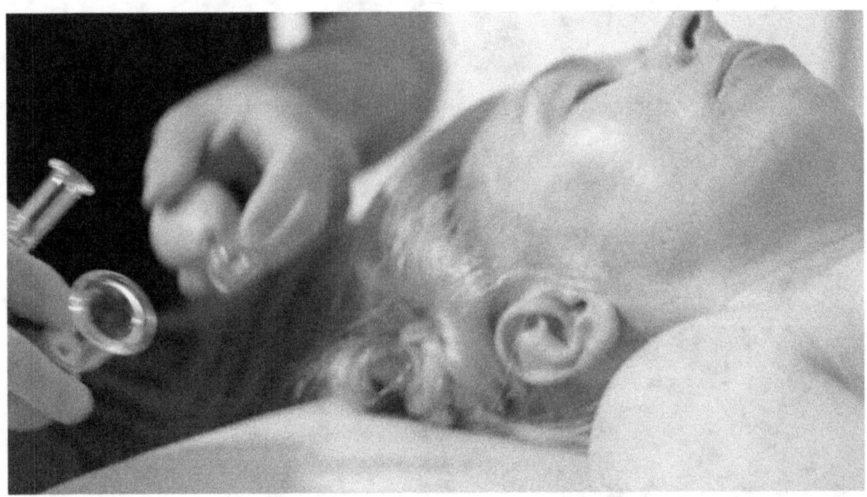

Begin by applying a small amount of oil to the client's face and lightly massaging it evenly.

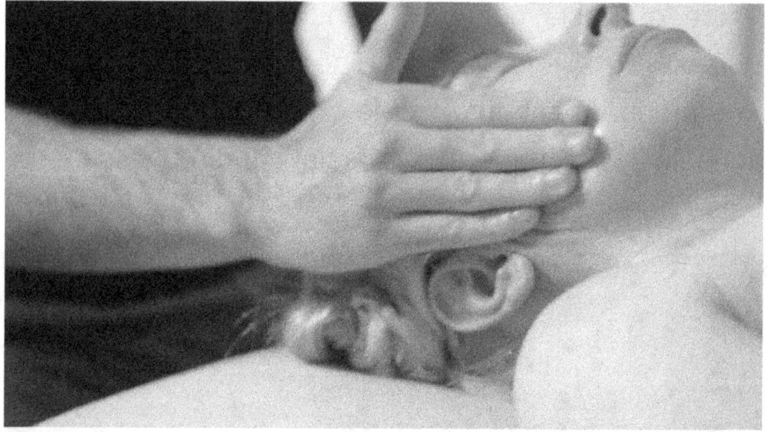

Make sure to apply enough oil so that when you apply the cups to the skin, it's nice and moist.

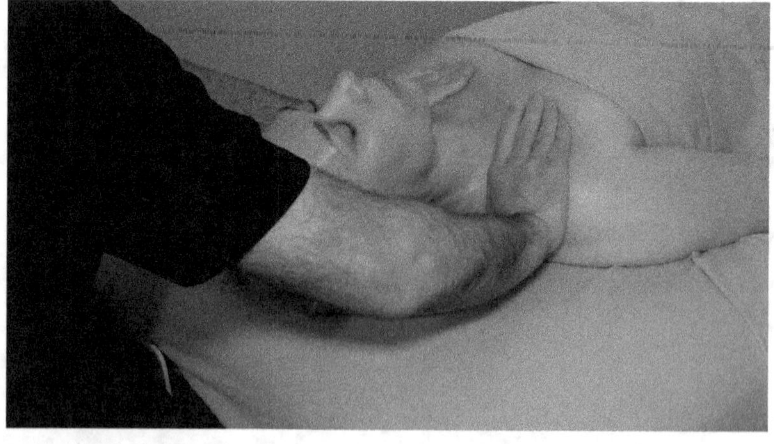

NOTE: Don't forget the décolleté (women's neckline).

Step 1: Lymphatic Drainage

Equipment needed: large-size facial cup.

Turn the client's face 45 degrees to the left, as you will begin with the right side of the face.

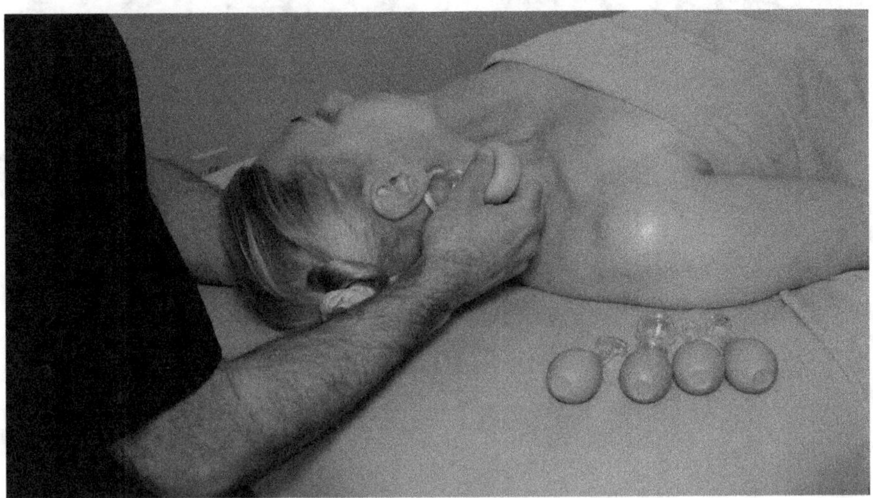

Begin with the suction release (SR) method down the sternocleidomastoid (SCM) on the lateral side of the neck by pinching the bulb, which creates a suction lifting the skin. Gently hold the suction for one to three seconds and then release by squeezing the bulb again.

NOTE: Make sure *not* to glide across the carotid artery or jugular vein when doing the SR down the SCM.

Cupping Massage
M A S T E R Y

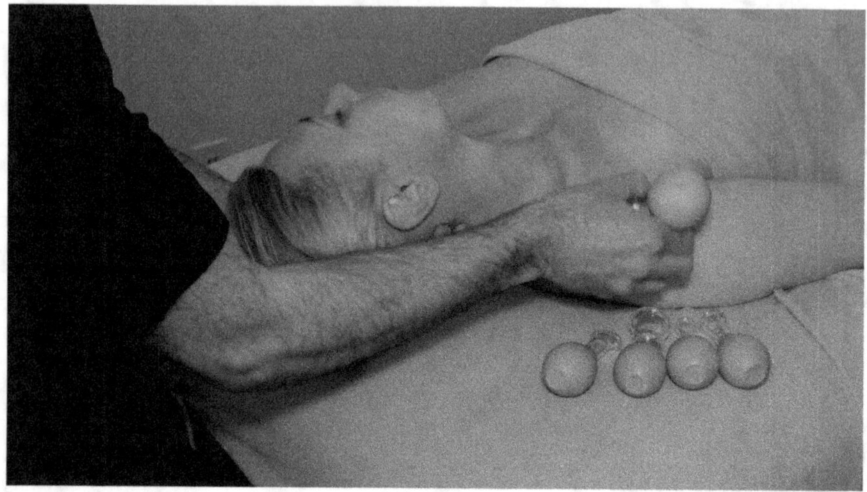

Do the SR method down the length of the SCM all the way to the clavicle and SR across the subclavius muscle (which is below the clavicles) toward the armpits, draining toward the axillary duct.

Cupping Massage
M A S T E R Y

Step 2: Jawline

Equipment needed: large-size or medium-size facial cup.

Starting right below the middle of the jawline, gently glide the cup along the jawline toward the parotid region (which is right below the ear and in front of the SCM).

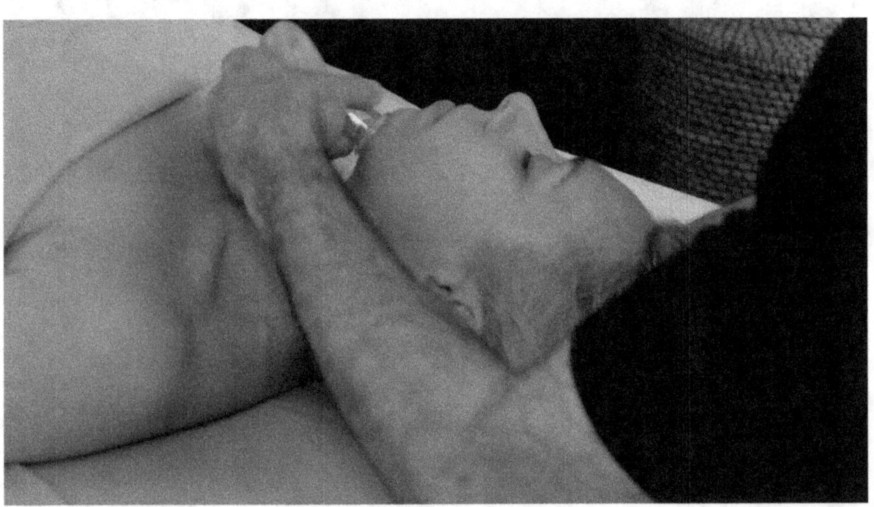

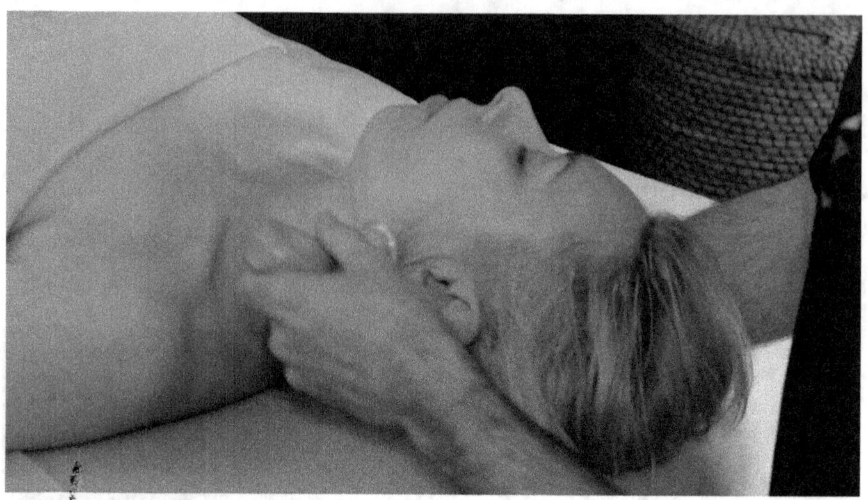

Do three sets of 10 passes. Each pass should gradually get higher up (superior) until the third set is directly on the jawline itself.

Next, you want to drain by suction releasing from the parotid down the SCM to the clavicle, and then across the subclavius toward the axillary duct.

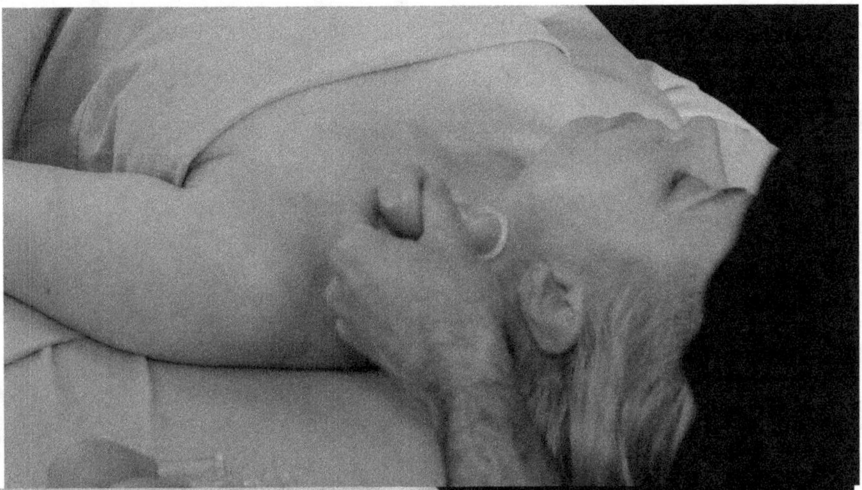

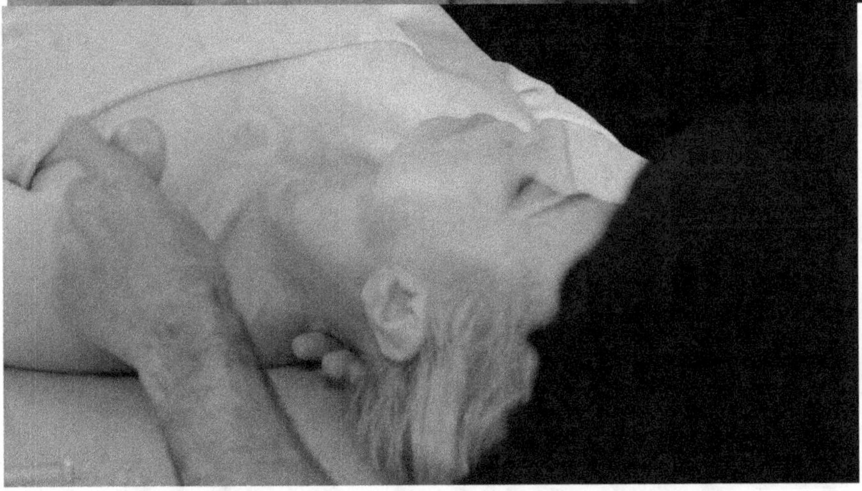

Step 3: Cheeks

Equipment needed: medium-size and large-size facial cups.

Suction and glide from right above the jawline toward the temporal mandibular joint (TMJ). Do this 10 times.

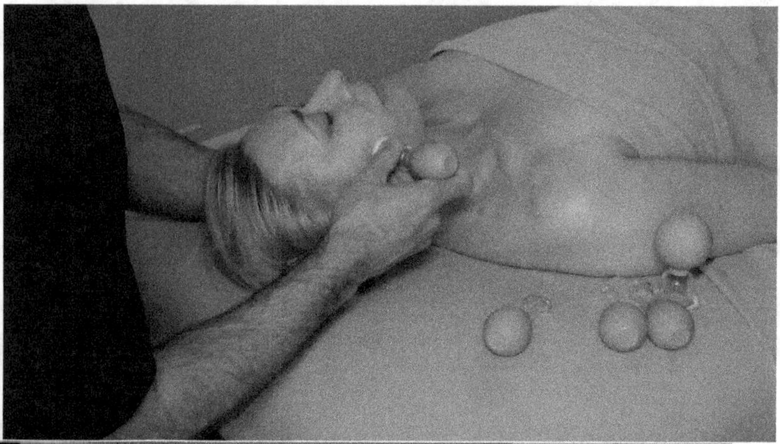

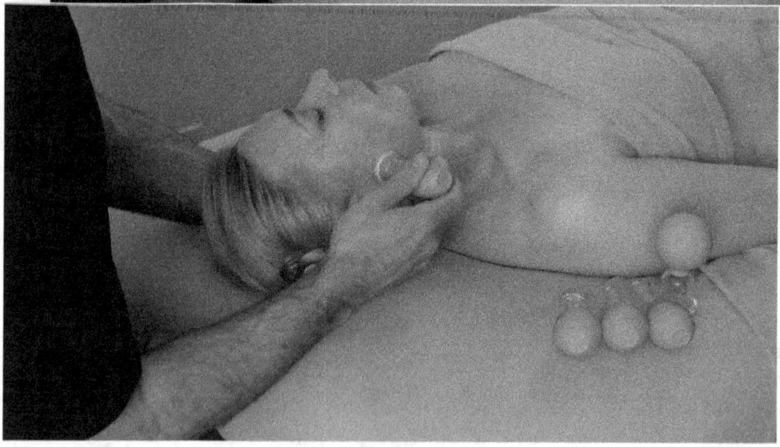

Next, drain by suction releasing from the parotid down the SCM to the clavicle, and then across the subclavius toward the axillary duct. Do this 10 times.

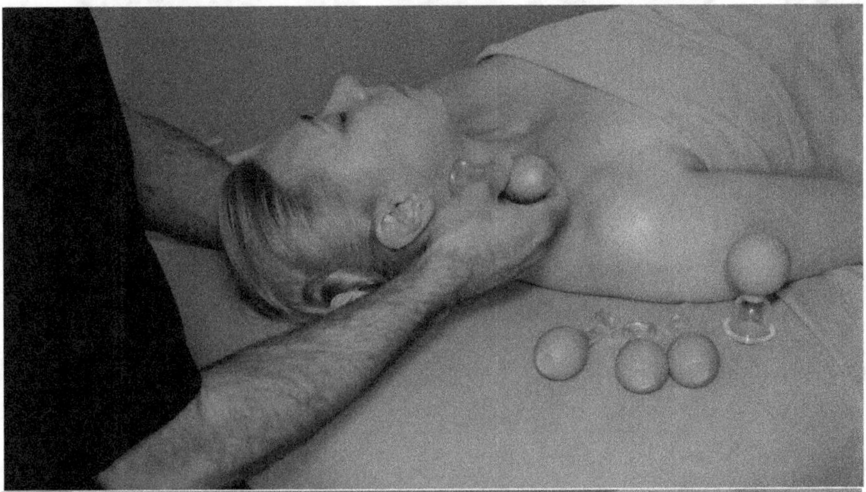

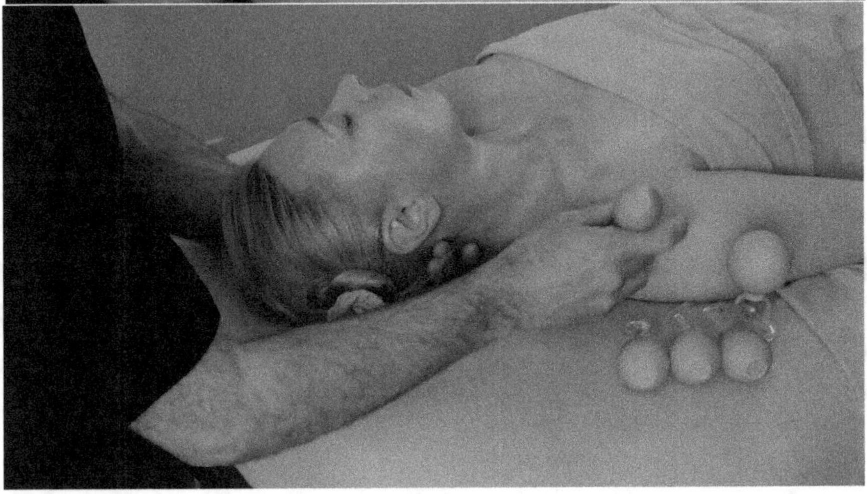

Suction and glide from the side of the mouth across the cheeks to the TMJ. Do this 10 times.

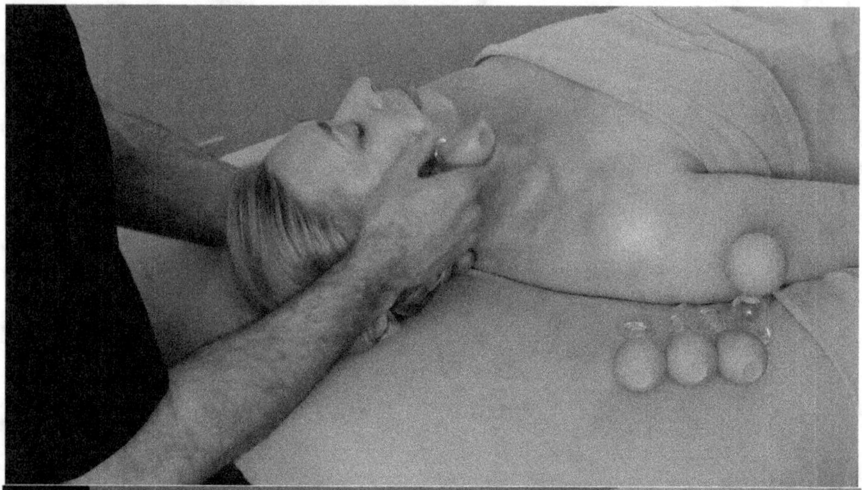

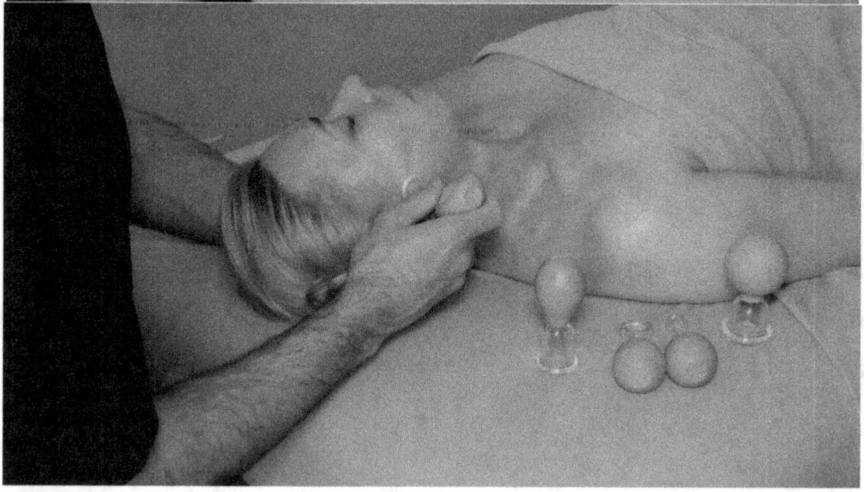

Last, drain by suctioning down the SCM, across the subclavius toward the axillary duct. Do this 10 times.

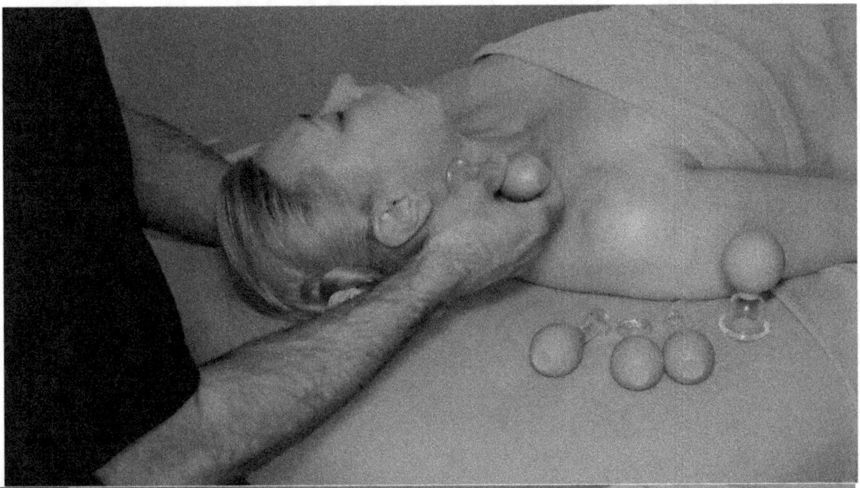

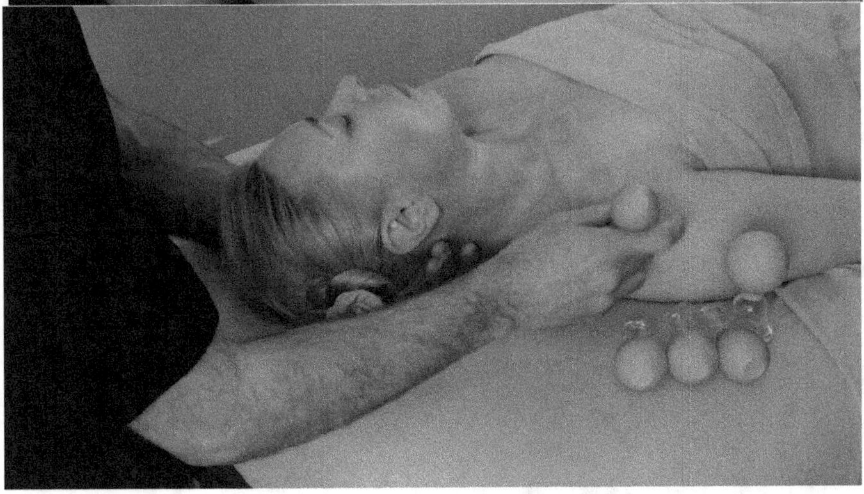

Step 4: Around the Mouth

Equipment needed: medium-size facial cup.

Switch to the medium-size facial cup. SR around the mouth. Do one to two full circles around the mouth.

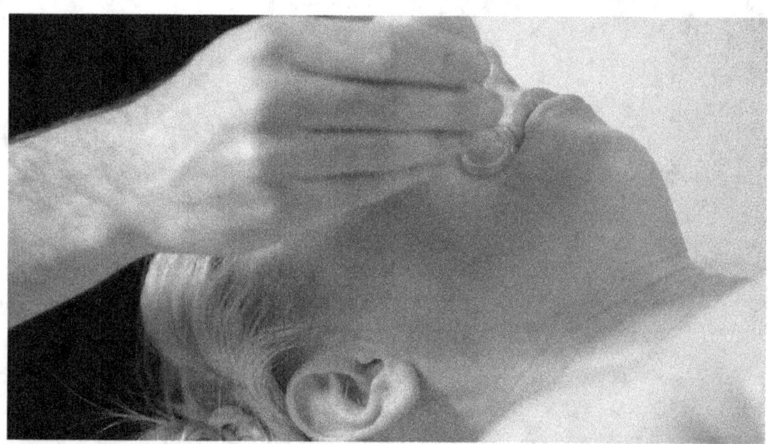

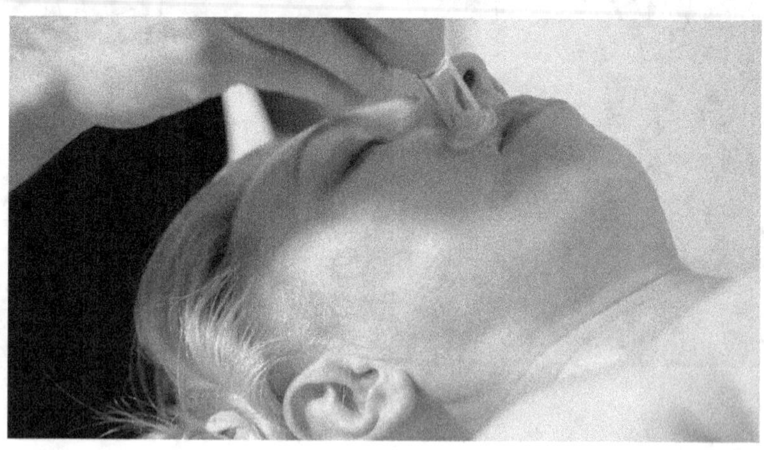

Cupping Massage
MASTERY

Spend a little extra time suctioning and dragging the expression lines around the mouth.

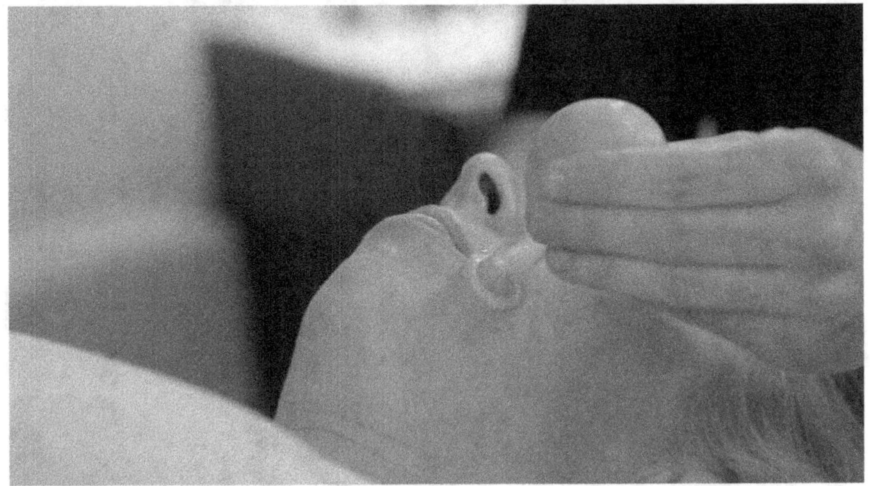

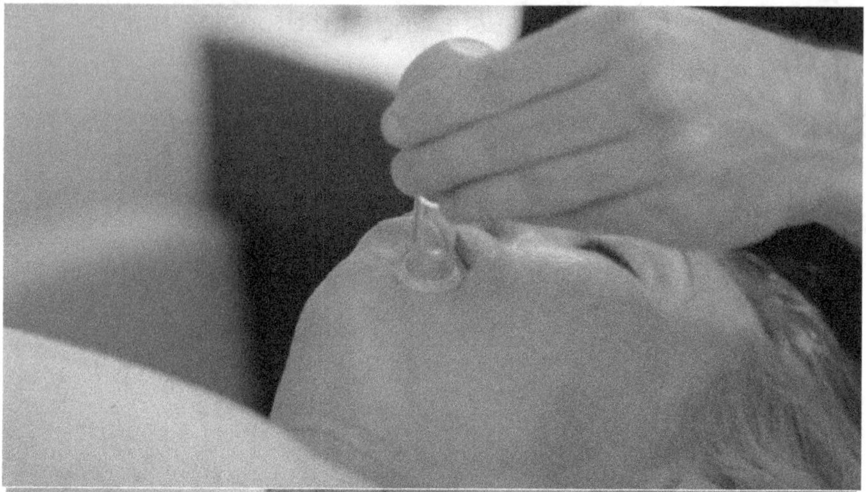

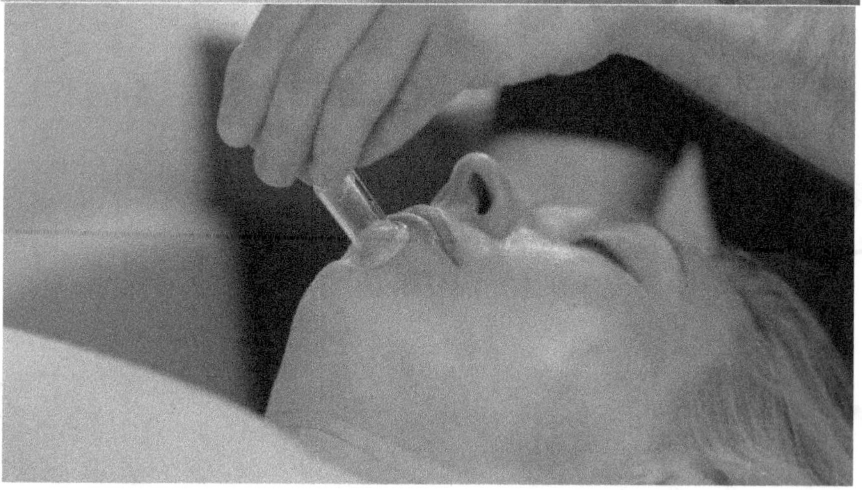

Cupping Massage
MASTERY

Step 5: Plump the Lips

Equipment needed: large-size facial cup.

Suction the lips, lift and hold for five seconds, and then release the lips. Divide the treatment in three sections: left, middle, right.

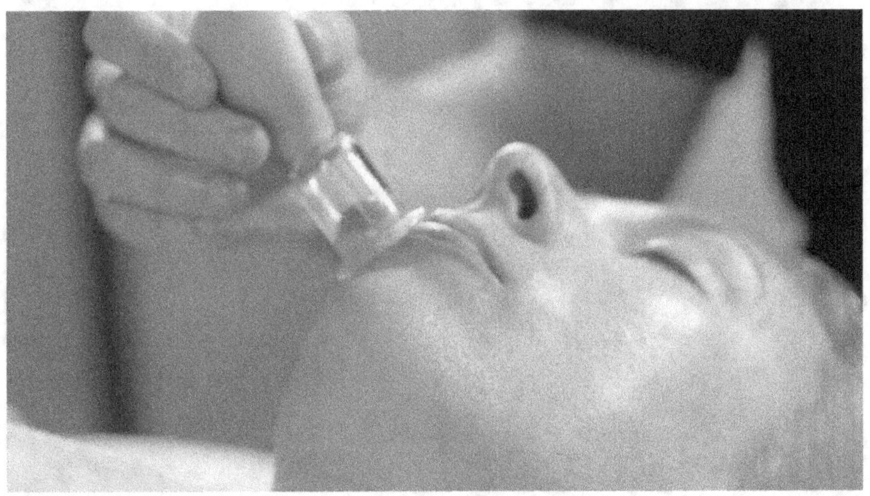

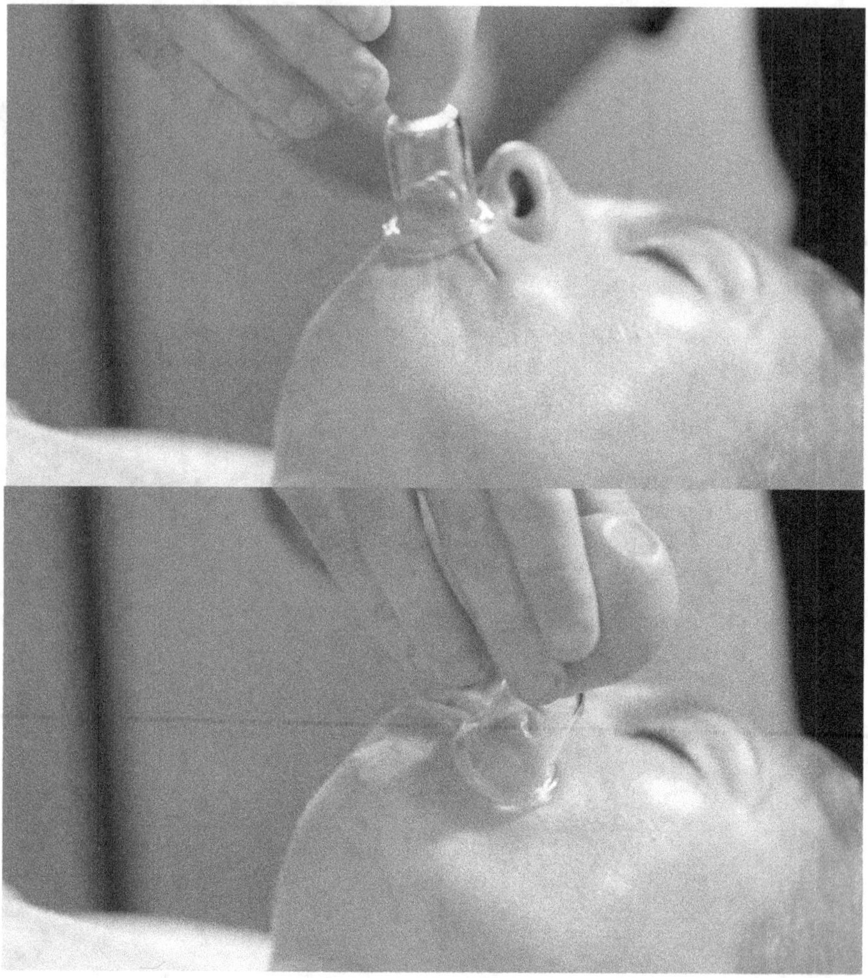

Finish plumping the lips by draining and suctioning down the SCM, across the subclavius toward the axillary duct. Do this 10 times.

Step 6: Sides of Nose

Equipment needed: oval facial cup and small-size facial cup.

The Nostrils

Using the oval facial cup, SR the nostrils five times.

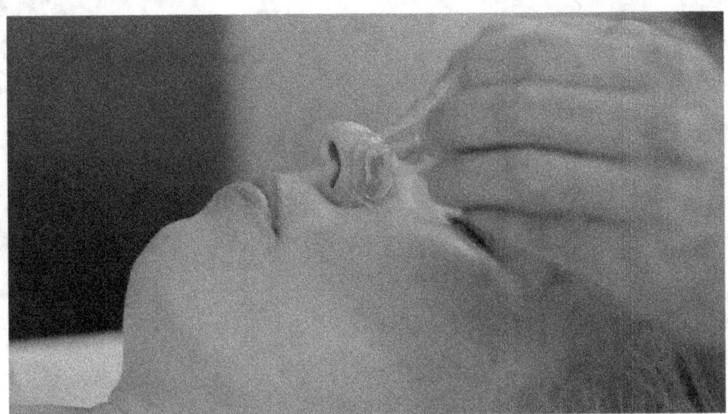

While you suction one nostril, use the index finger of your non-cupping hand to support the opposite side of the nose.

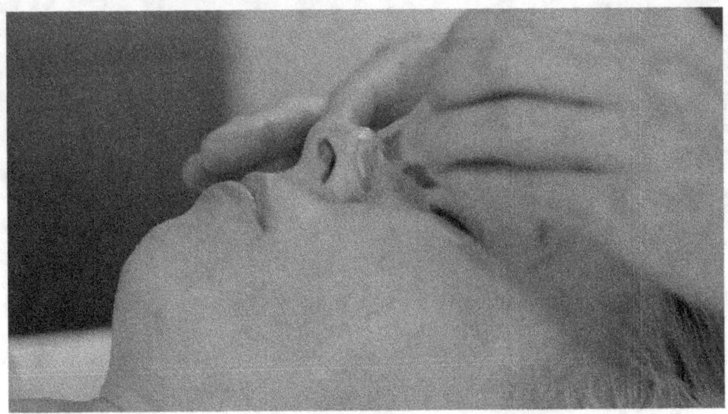

The Tip of the Nose

SR the tip of the nose five times. If the oblong cup doesn't fit well, drop down a size to a smaller size cup.

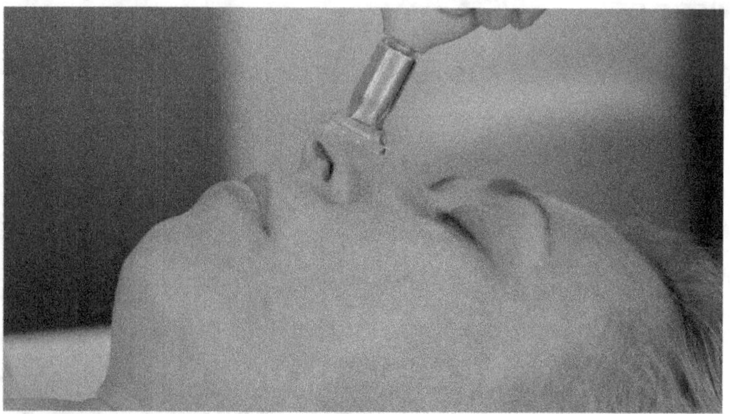

The Bridge of the Nose

SR the bridge of the nose five times.

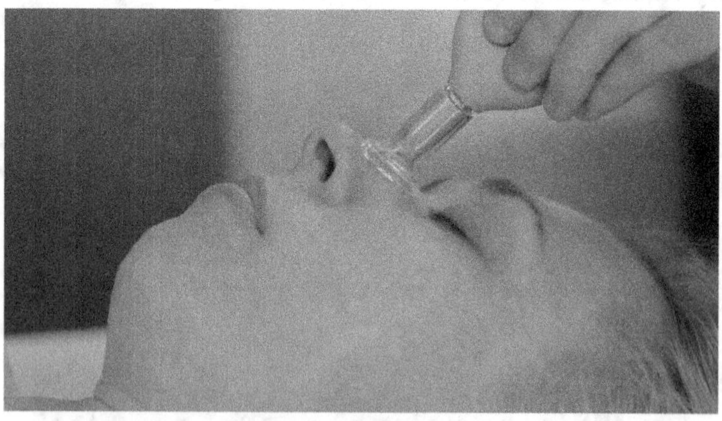

The Sides of the Nose

SR the side of the nose (the side of the face you're working on) five times.

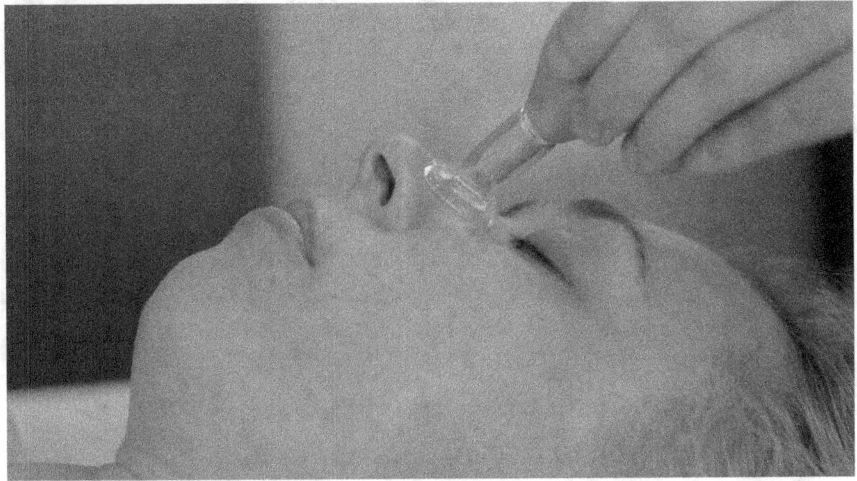

When suctioning the side of the nose, it helps to use your other hand's index finger to support the opposite side of the nose.

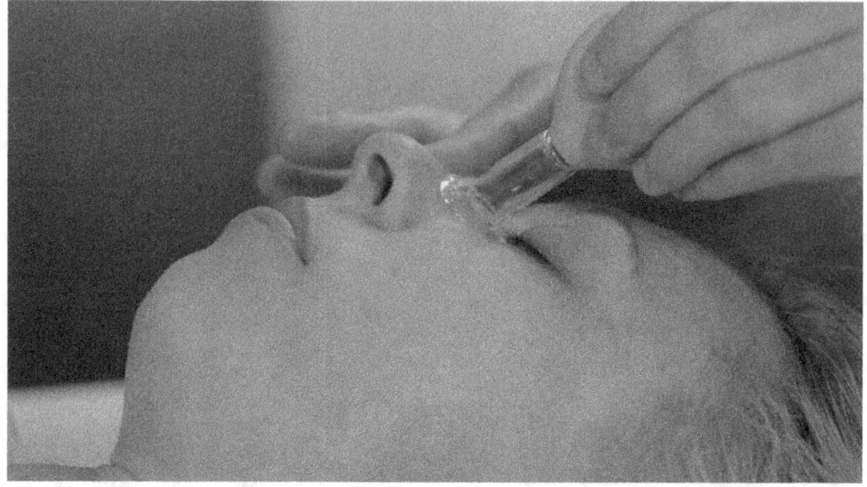

Drain by dragging the cup down the cheek and then switch to the medium-size cup. SR down the SCM, across the subclavius toward the axillary duct. Do this 10 times.

Now repeat the entire sequence using the small-size facial cup.

The Nostrils

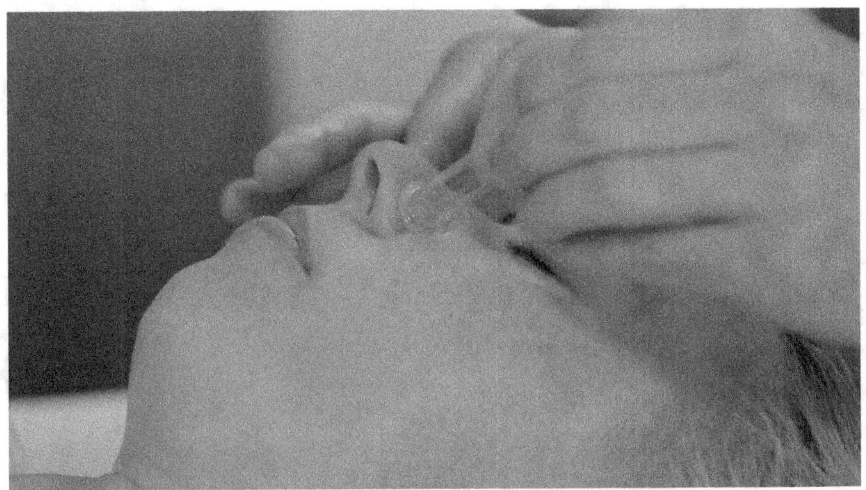

The Tip of the Nose

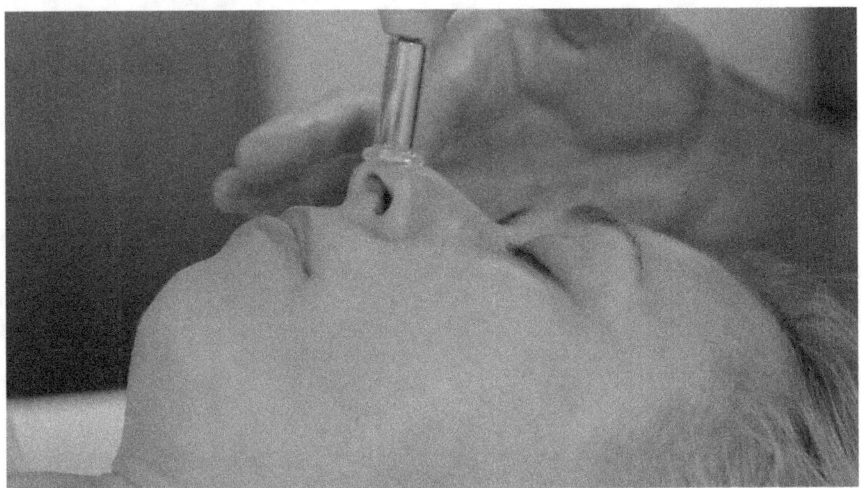

The Sides of the Nose

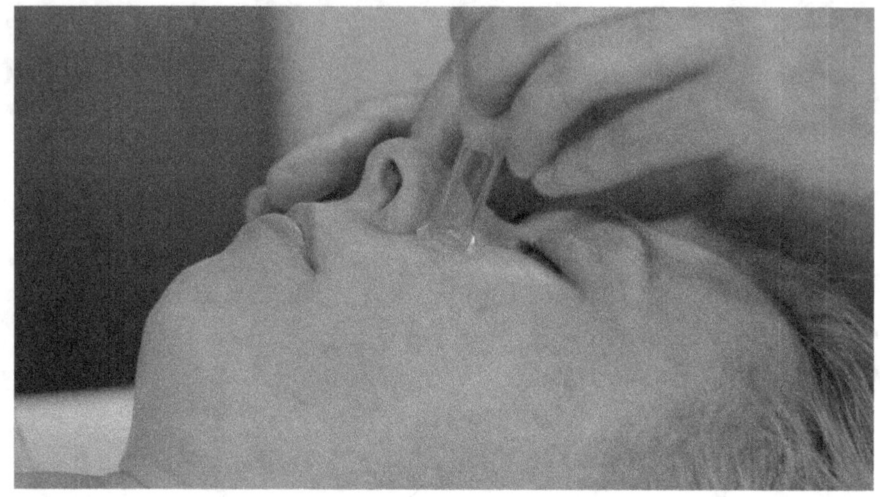

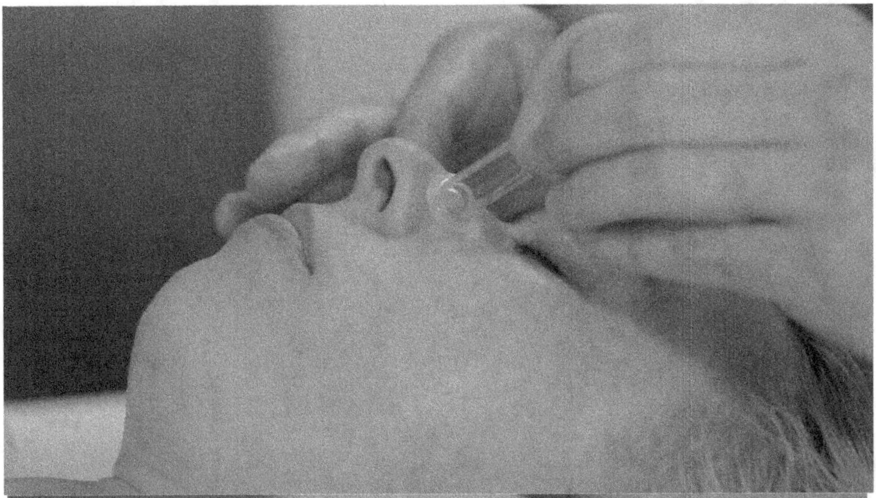

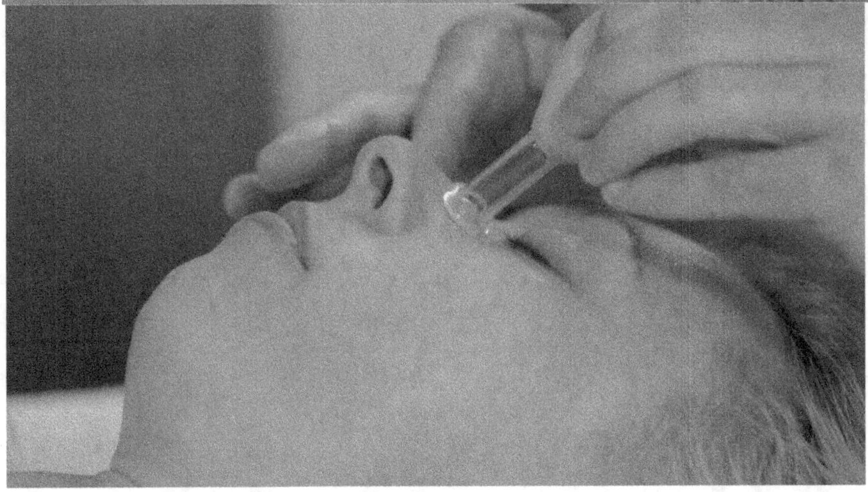

Cupping Massage
M A S T E R Y

Step 7: Around the Eyes

Equipment needed: small-size or oval facial cup.

Below the Eye

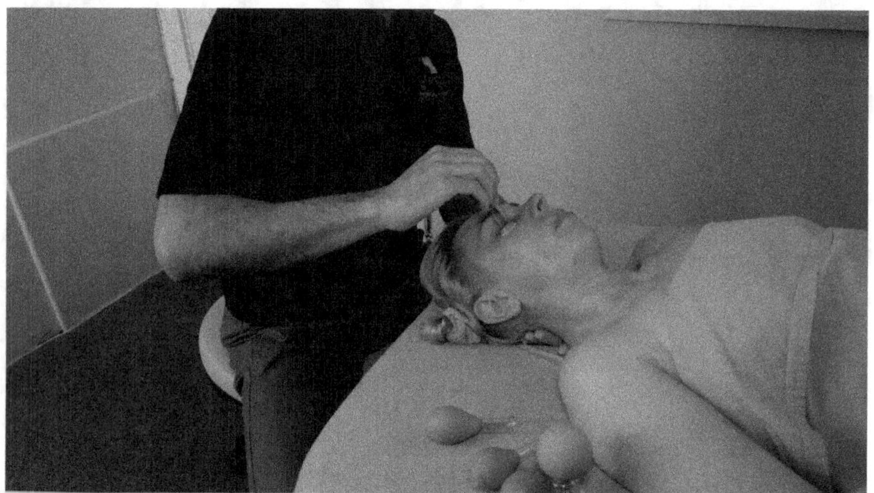

Gently place the cup at the *bottom of the orbital ridge* and get as close as you can to the eyelid, and then SR three times to the corner of the eye. Do three sets.

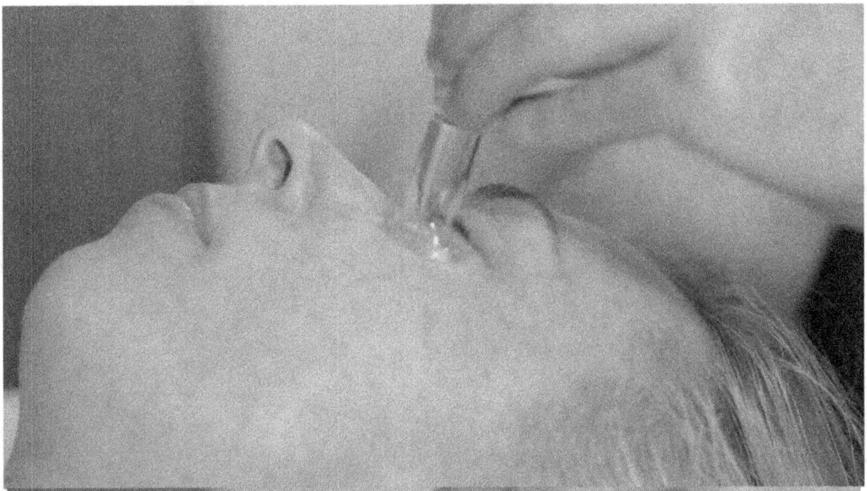

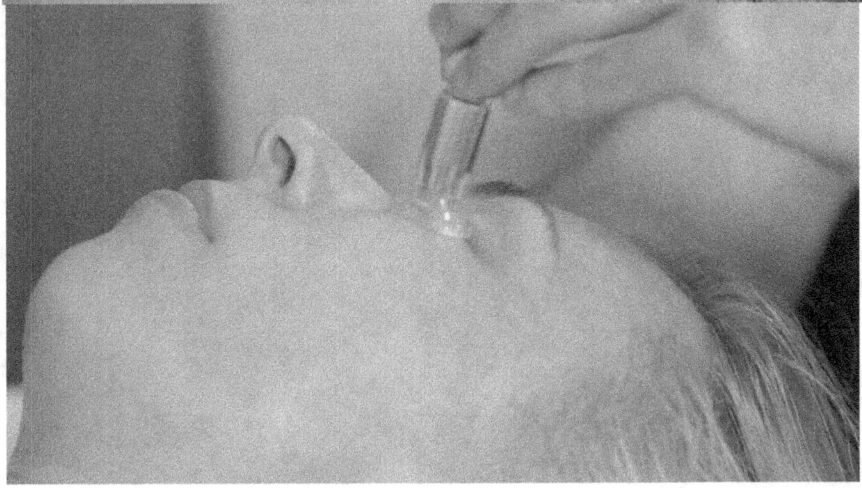

Cupping Massage
MASTERY

Cupping Massage
MASTERY

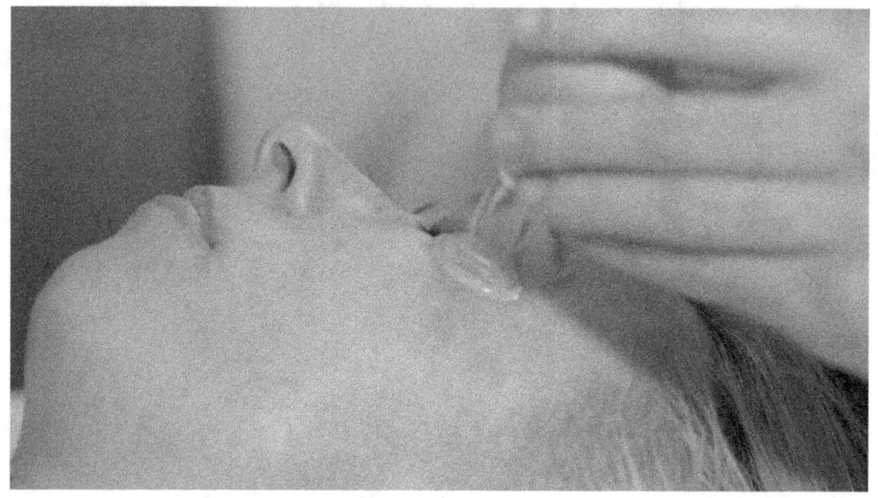

Above the Eye

Now do the *top of the orbital ridge* and get as close as you can to the eyelid, and then SR three times to the corner of the eye. Do three sets.

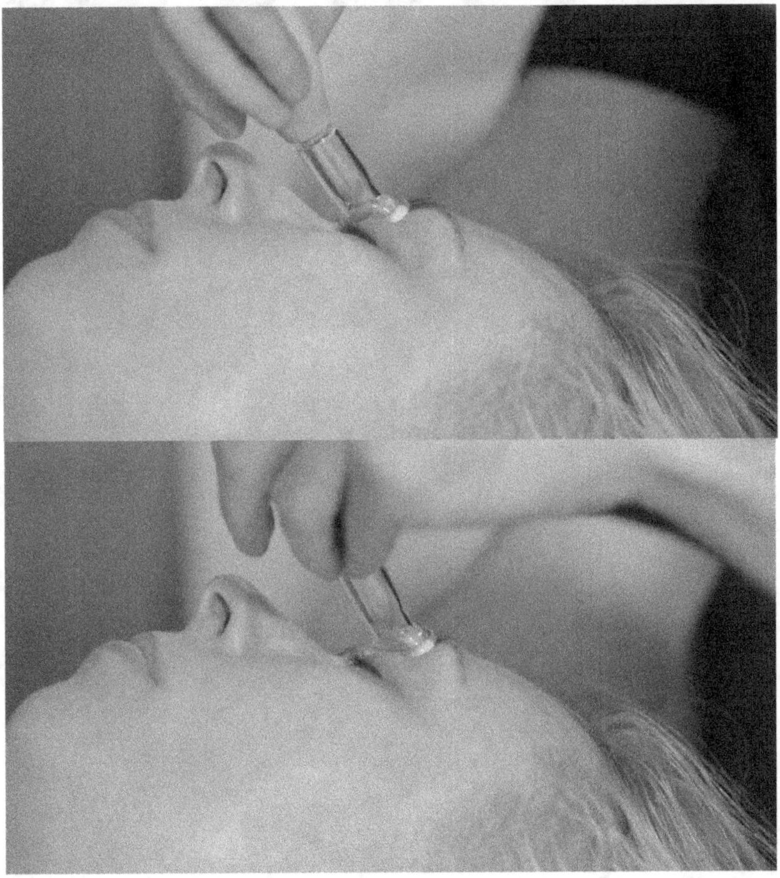

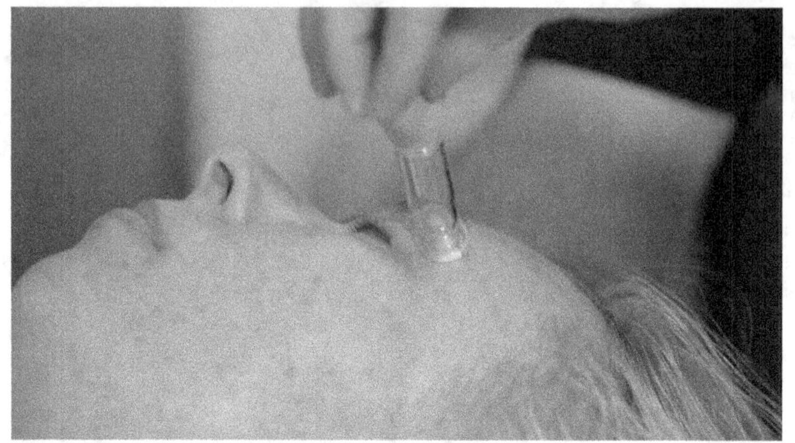

Crow's Feet

SR the side of the eyes (crow's feet) three times. Use a sweeping or flicking movement. Do three sets.

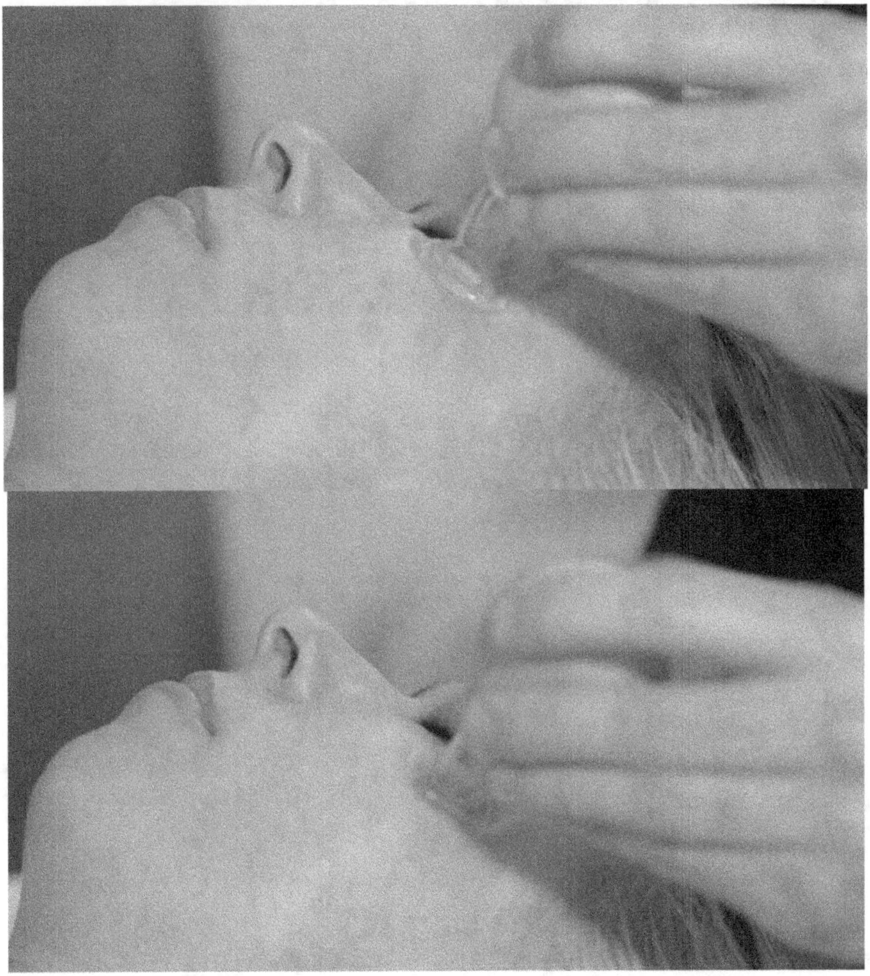

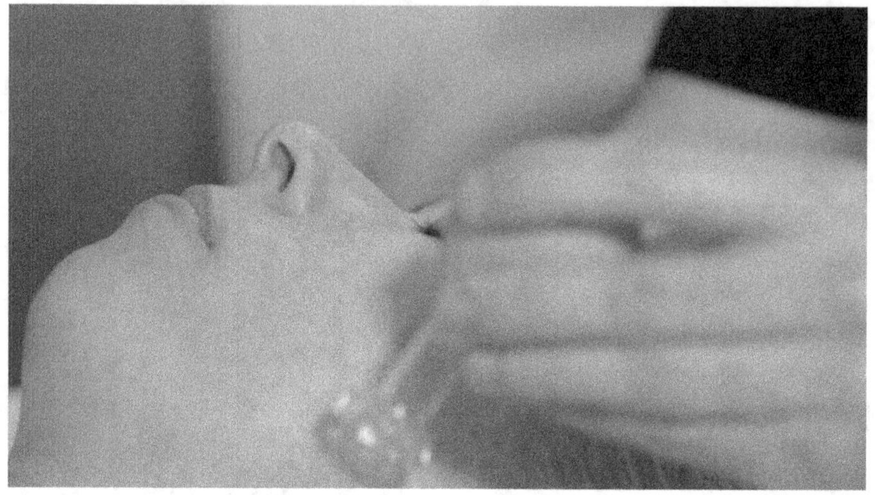

Crow's Feet (Wide Shot)

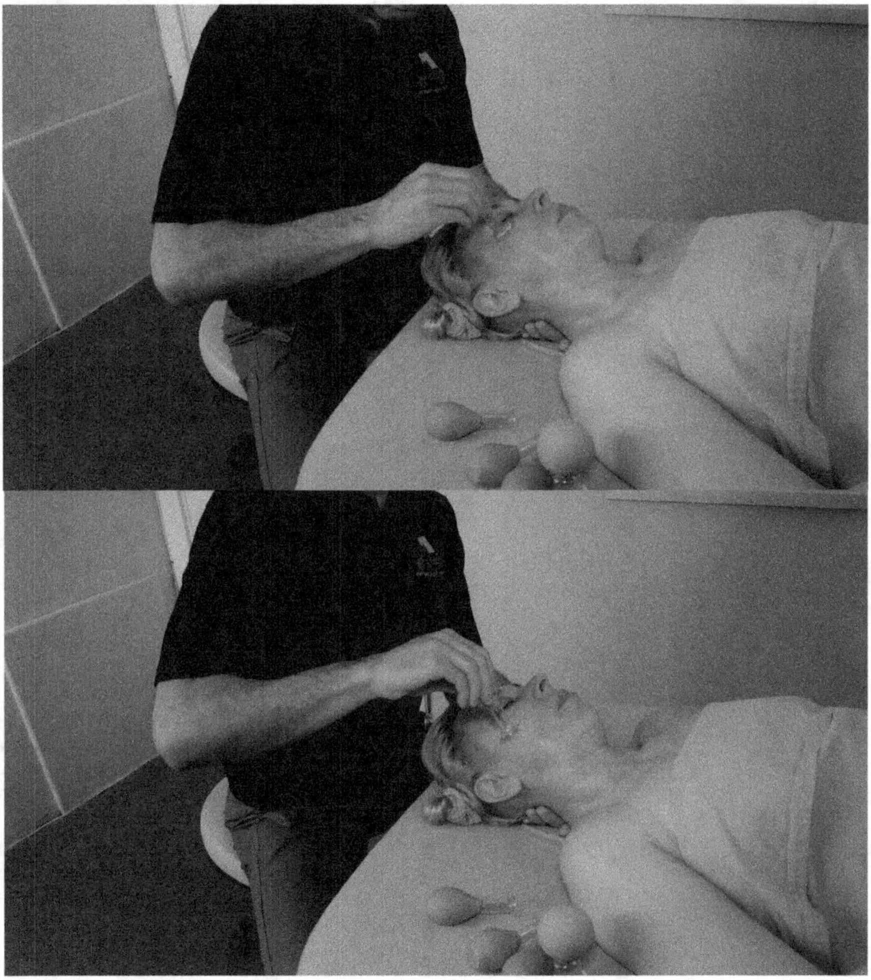

Finish and Drain

Using the large-size facial cup, suction and gently drag from the side of the eye, across the TMJ to the parotid, and then SR down the SCM, across the subclavius toward the axillary duct. Do this 10 times.

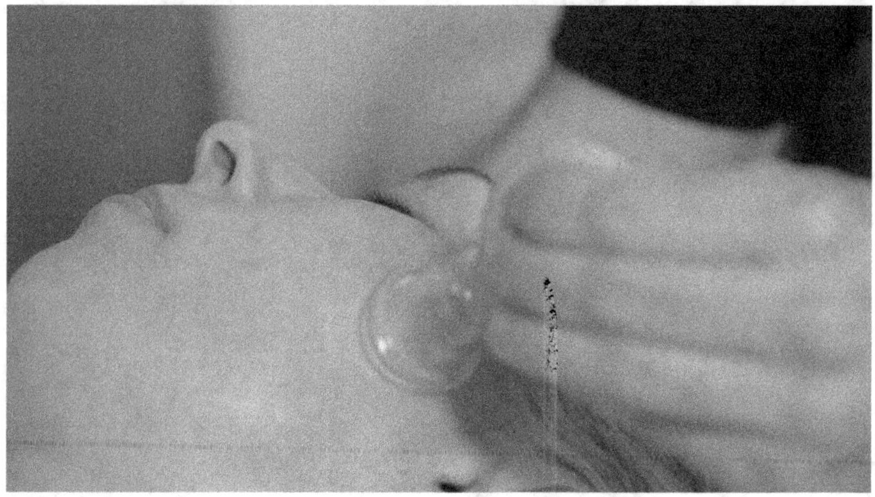

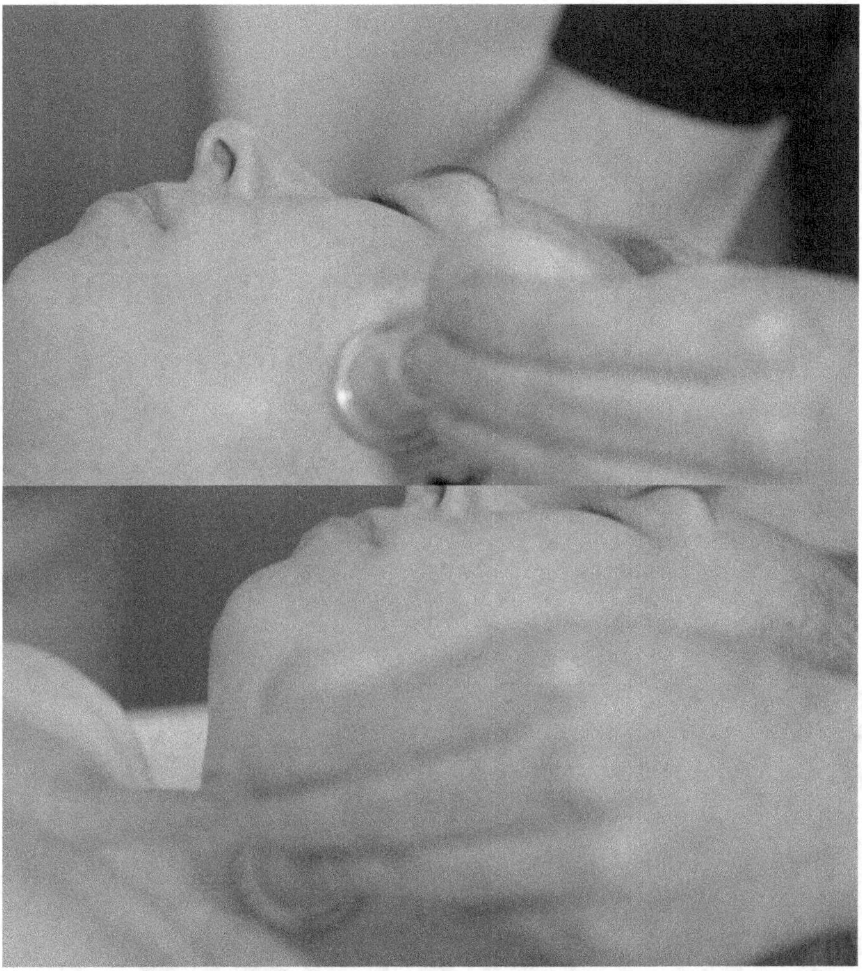

Cupping Massage
MASTERY

Step 8: Frown Lines and Forehead

Equipment needed: large-size facial cup.

SR the frown lines between the eyebrows using the medium-size cup. Each SR should last approximately five seconds.

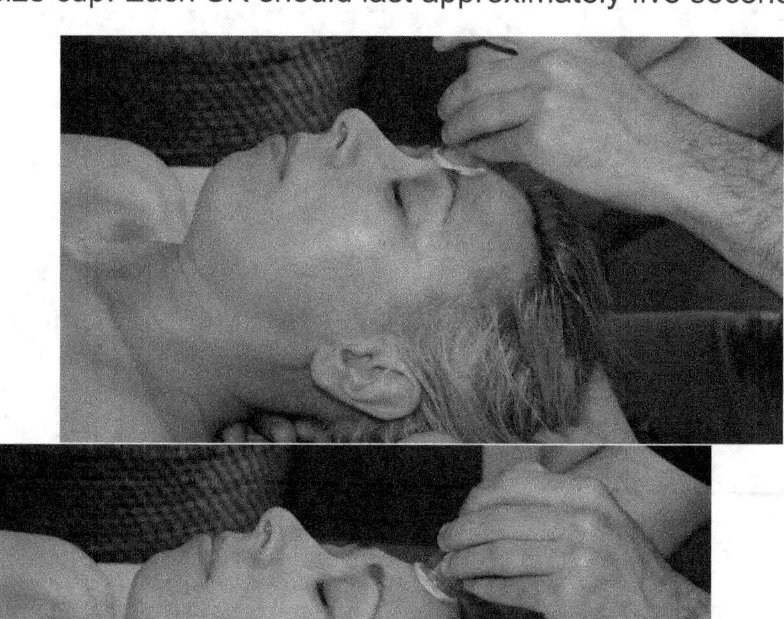

Using the large-size oval cup, suction and glide vertically from the eyebrows to the hairline. Do three sets of three passes.

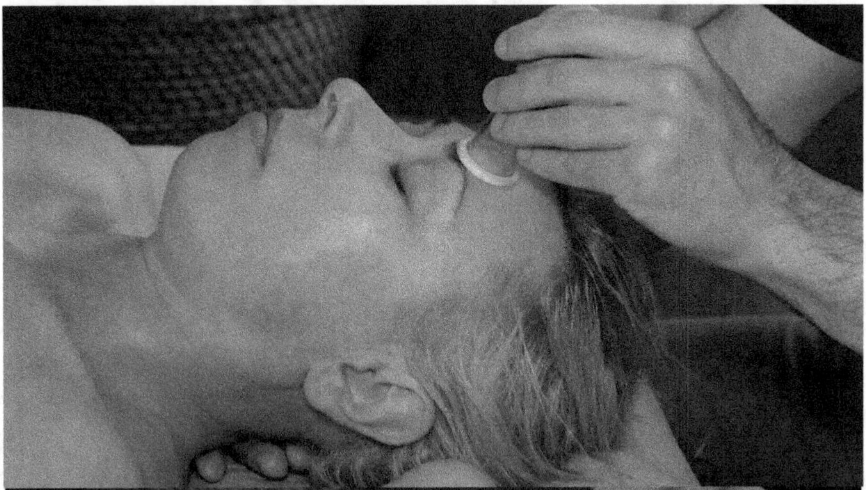

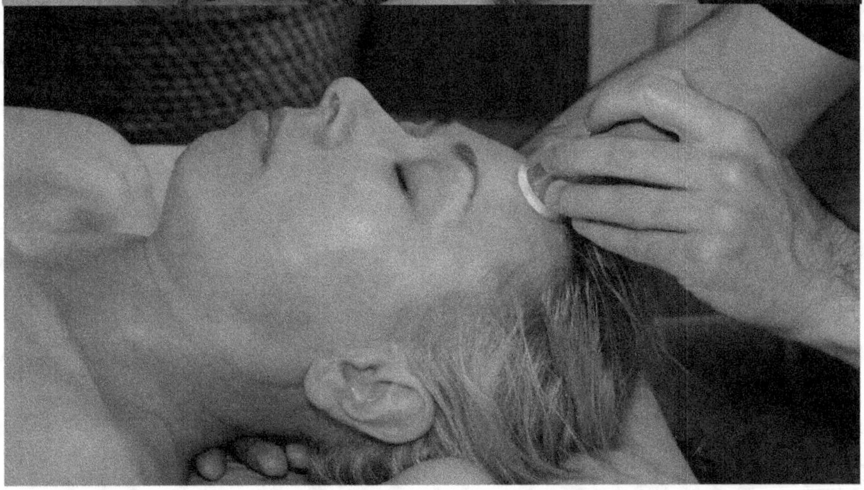

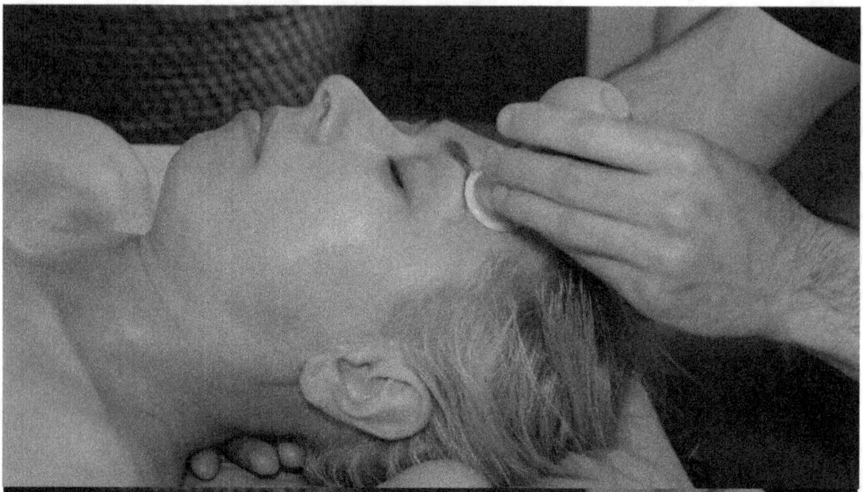

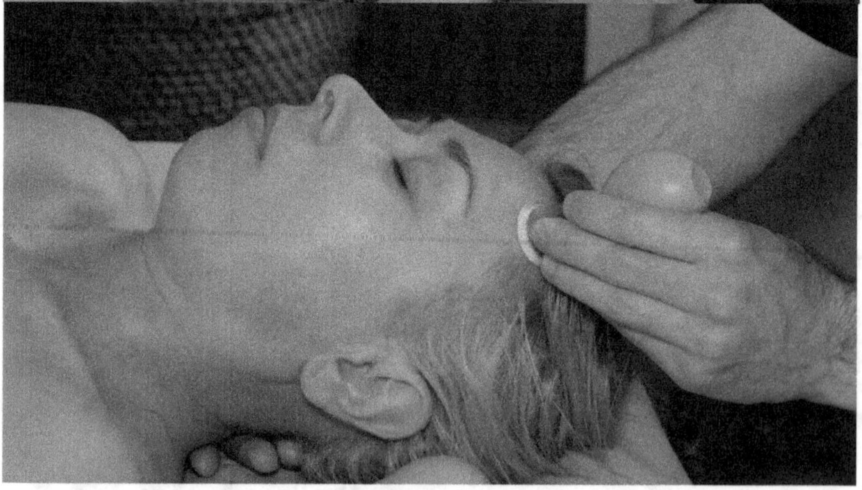

Now, suction and glide horizontally across the forehead toward the temples. Do three sets of three passes covering the entire forehead from above the eyebrows to the hairline.

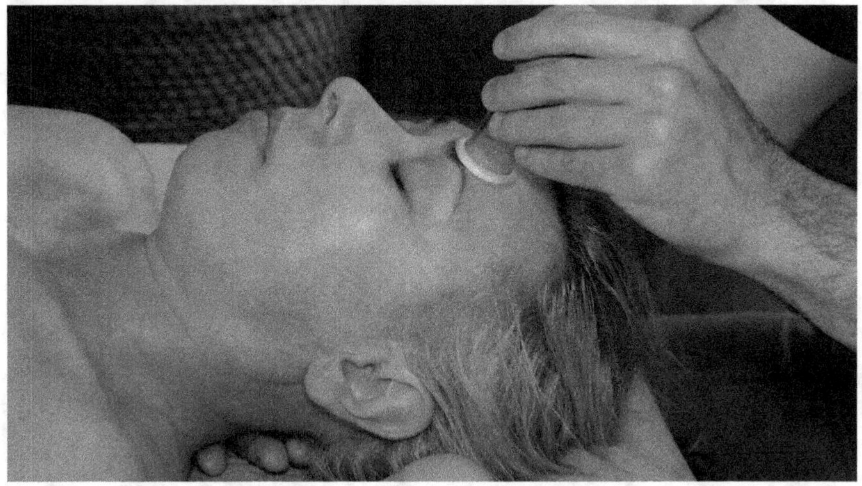

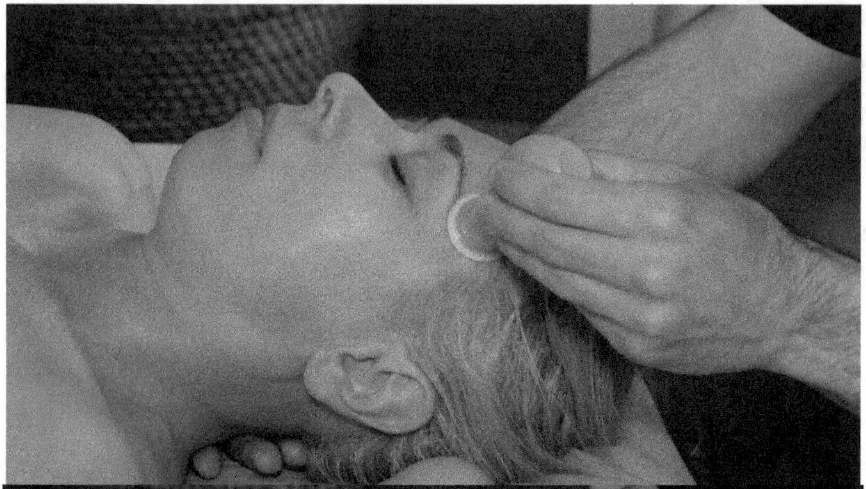

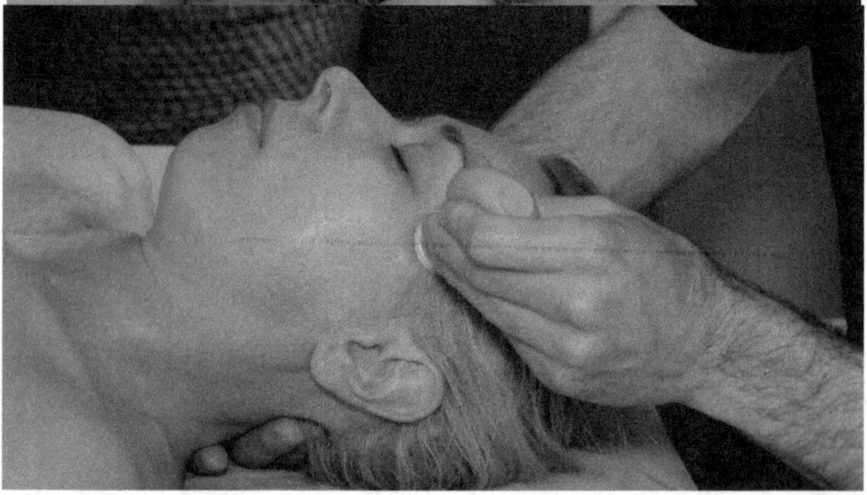

Cupping Massage
MASTERY

Drain from temples down the TMJ to the parotid, and then SR down the SCM, across the subclavius toward the axillary duct. Do this 10 times.

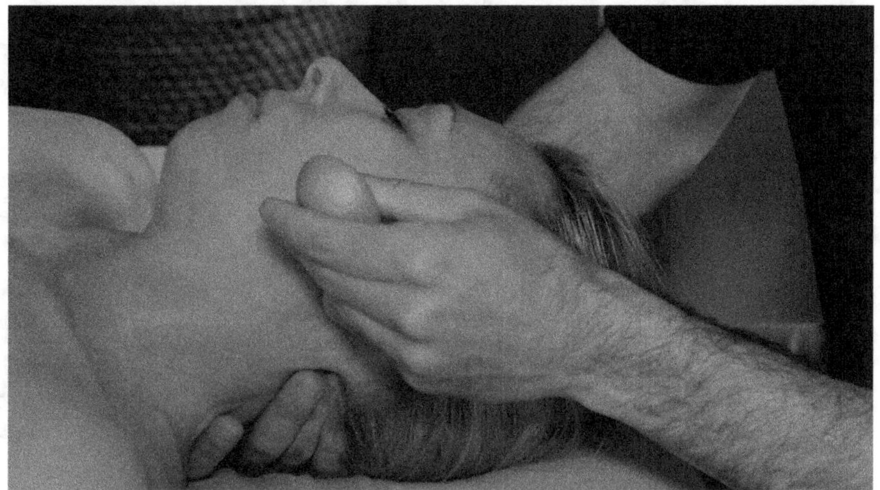

Cupping Massage
M A S T E R Y

Step 9: Eyebrows

Equipment needed: small-size and medium-size facial cup.

SR directly over and above the eyebrows. Do three sets of three passes.

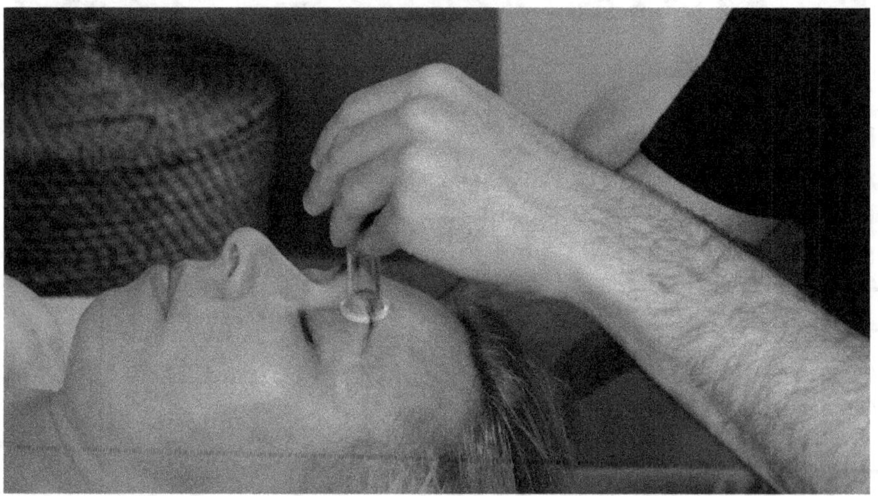

Drain from the temples down the TMJ to the parotid, and then SR down the SCM, across the subclavius toward the axillary duct. Do this 10 times.

Now repeat the entire sequence on the other side of the face.

Step 10: Finishing Strokes

After you've finished the facial cupping routine, perform a gentle facial massage to end the session.

1. Spread the Forehead

Do this two times.

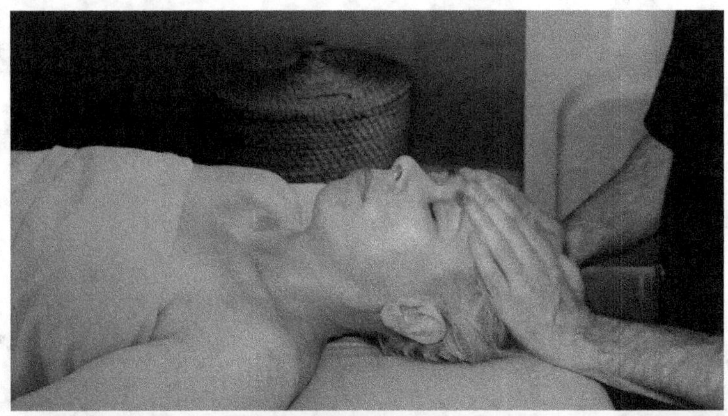

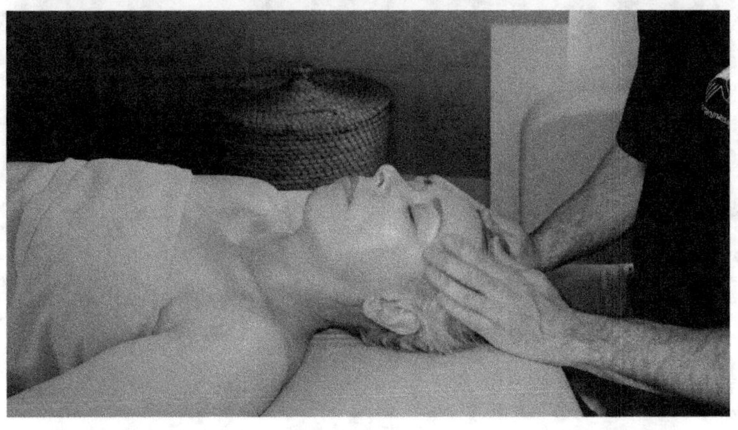

2. Trace the Cheek Line

Do this one time.

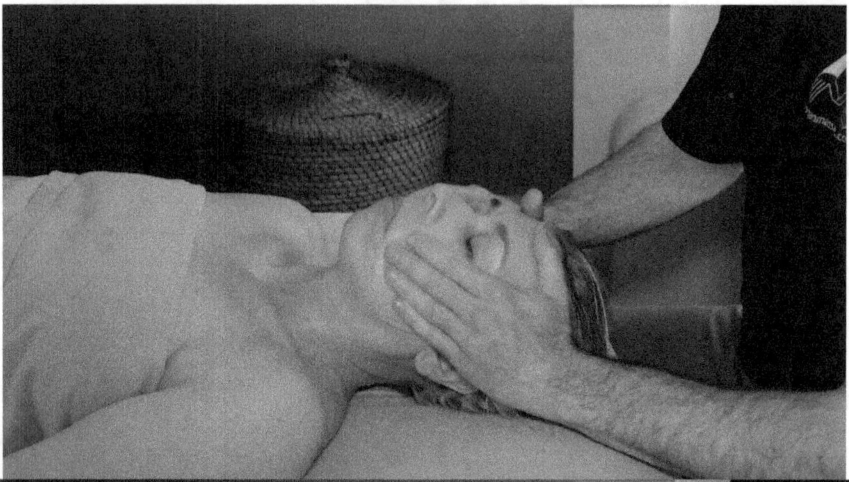

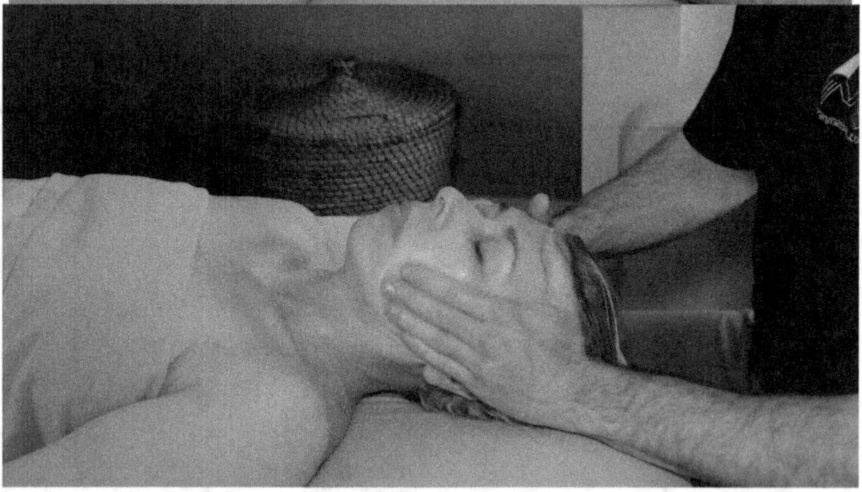

3. Trace the Jawline

Do this one time.

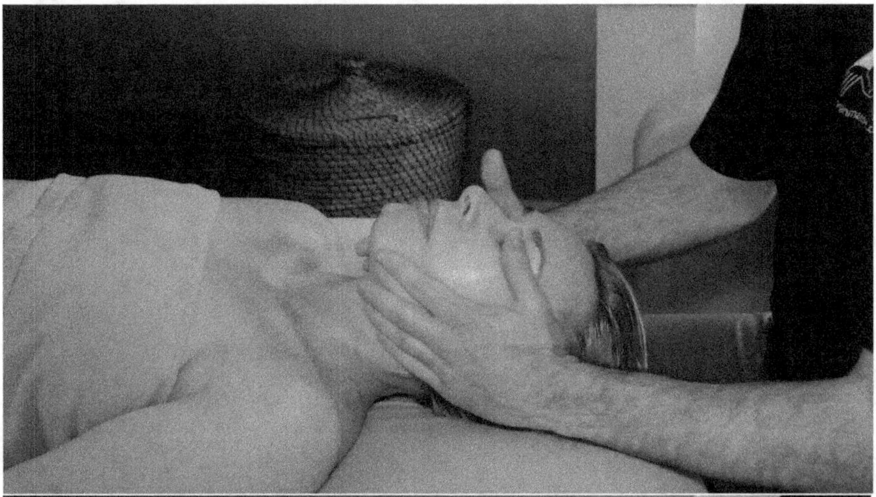

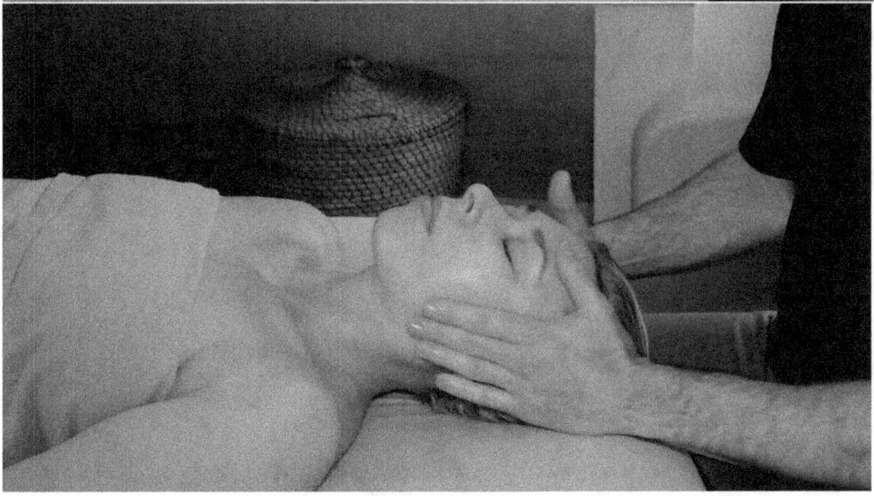

4. Spreading the Chest

Do this one time.

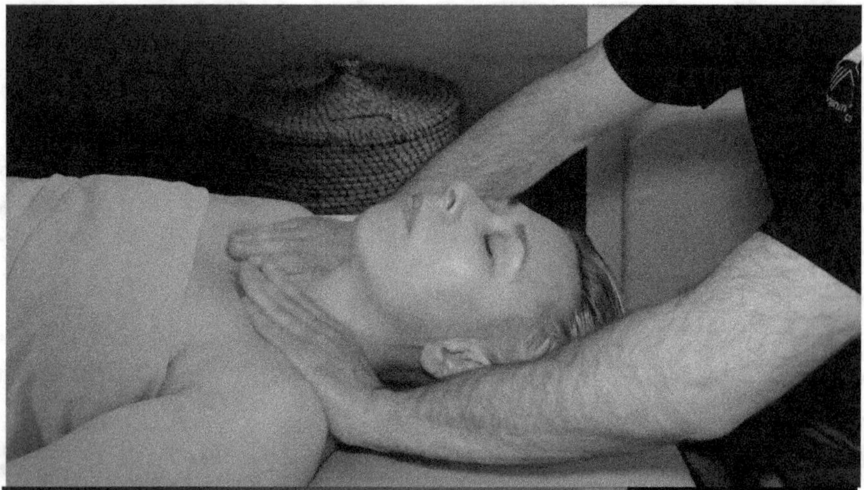

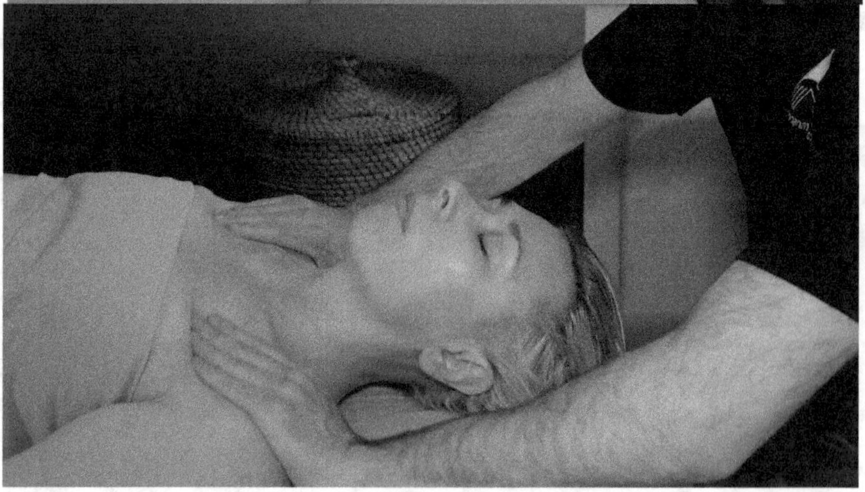

5. Neck Squeeze

Do this one time (or as many times as you'd like; this is a client favorite).

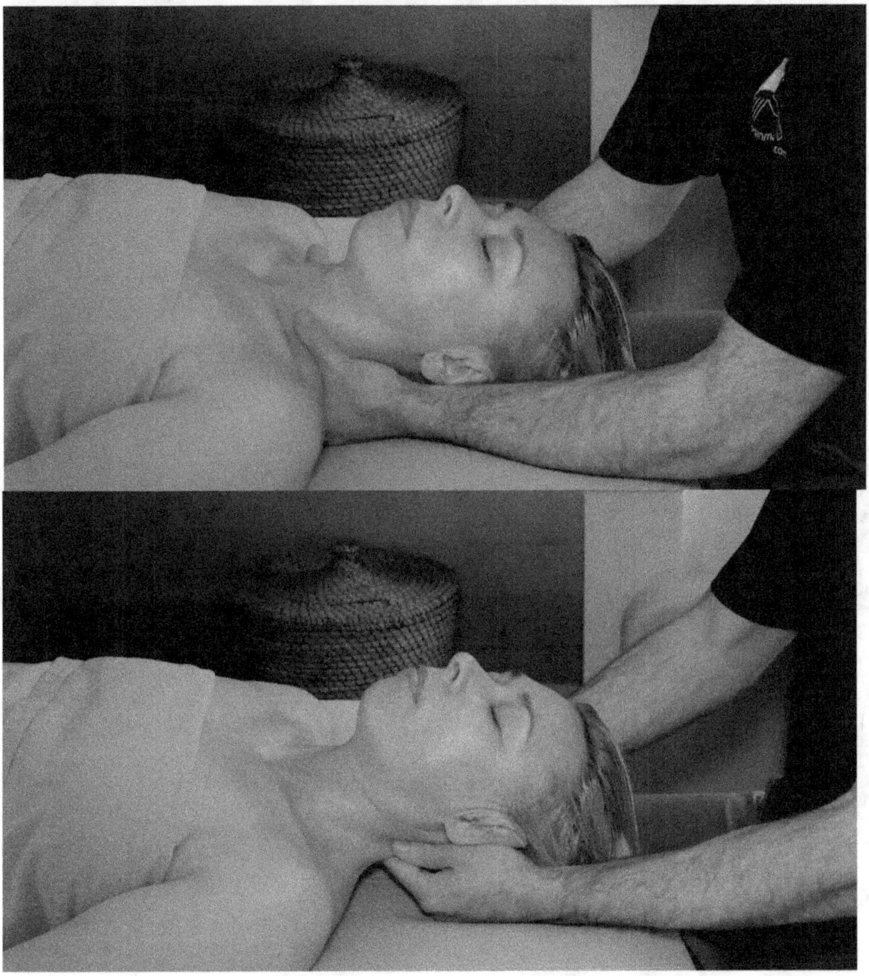

6. Trace the Jawline (Left Side)

Do this one time.

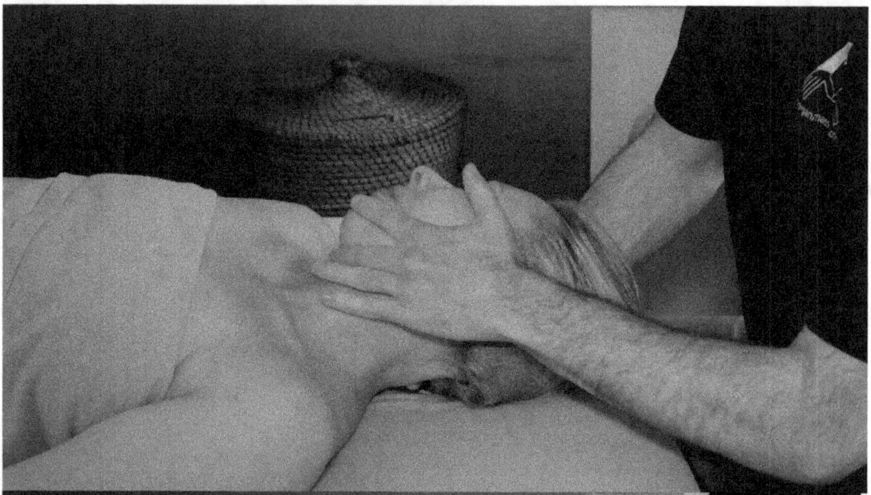

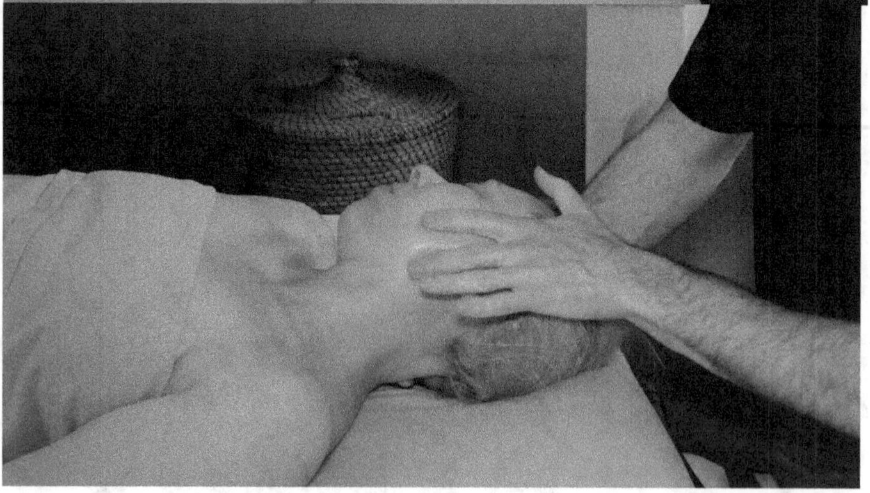

Cupping Massage
MASTERY

7. Trace the Cheek Line (Left Side)

Do this one time.

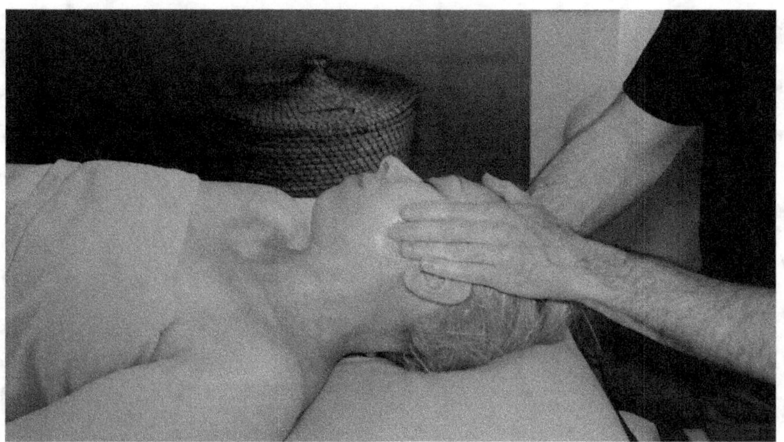

8. Spread the Forehead (Left Side)

Do this one time.

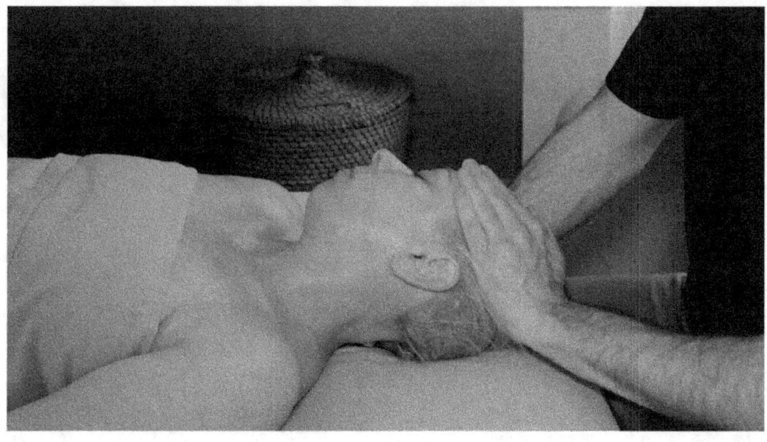

9. Spread the Pecs (Left Side)

Do this one time.

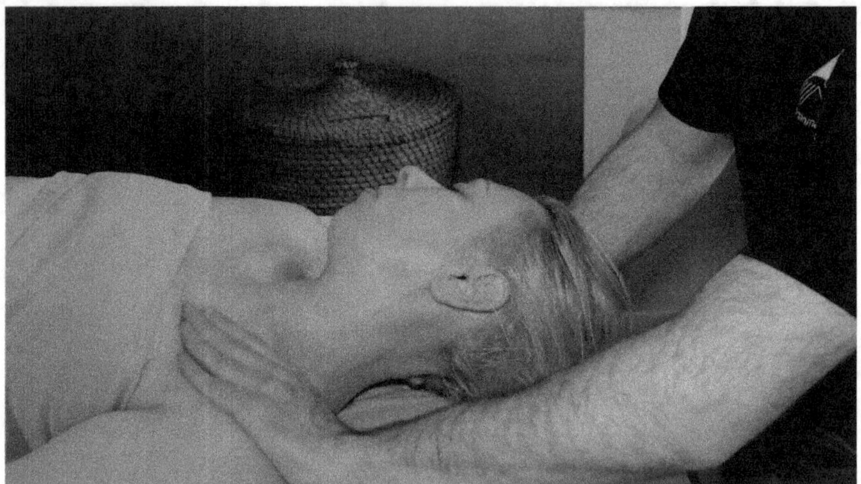

Repeat the finishing strokes on the right side.

Cupping Massage
M A S T E R Y

Helpful Tips

- Start with a clean face. Remove any makeup with a moist towelette or other makeup remover.

- Make sure to keep contact with the face with the other hand before touching the client's face with a cup.

- Always anchor the surrounding skin when gliding cups to prevent painful drag. Lift the cup slightly away from the skin to increase lymphatic activity.

- First-time clients: Have them sit up and examine the difference in a portable mirror after you've completed one side of the face. When they see how different the two sides of their face look, finish the treatment on the other side. With the client's permission, snap a photo with your smartphone to track before and after images.

- Use slower movements to drain more fluids. Faster movements are more stimulating for circulation and collagen/elastin building. Try beginning with slow, draining movements and progressively increase the speed over the three passes. The initial pass is slow, the second is at a medium speed, and the third pass is the fastest.

- For maximum facial rejuvenation results, it's recommended that the client comes in for facial cupping on a weekly basis for 6 to 12 consecutive weeks.

About the Author

Since becoming a professional massage therapist in 2000, Morgan Sutherland has consistently helped thousands of clients manage their pain with a combination of deep tissue work, cupping, and stretching. In 2002, he began a career-long tradition of continuing study by being trained in Tuina—the art of Chinese massage—at the world-famous Olympic Training Center in Beijing, China.

In 2004, Morgan became a certified orthopedic massage therapist, specializing in treating chronic pain and sports injuries. In 2005, Morgan took his fist cupping course and was immediately hooked. He mastered using the plastic Kangzhu Biomagnetic Chinese Cupping set and was amazed how easy the cups were to handle and apply.

In 2011, Morgan took more advanced cupping training and discovered silicone cups. The silicone cups literally became an extension of his hands, allowing him to seamlessly lift and release clients' muscle adhesions. Blending the silicone cupping into his deep tissue massage practice was effortless, and the majority of his client base raved about how much more effective his massage sessions have become.

When he's not helping clients manage their pain, he's writing blog posts about pain relief and self-care.

Website: www.cuppingmassagemastery.com

Email: info@cuppingmassagemastery.com

Other Books by Morgan Sutherland, L.M.T.

The Essential Lower Back Pain Exercise Guide: Treat Low Back Pain at Home in Twenty-One Days or Less

21 Yoga Exercises for Lower Back Pain: Stretching Lower Back Pain Away with Yoga

Reverse Bad Posture Exercises: Fix Neck, Back, and Shoulder Pain in Just 15 Minutes Per Day

Best Treatment for Sciatica Pain: Relieve Sciatica Symptoms, Piriformis Muscle Pain, and SI Joint Pain in Just 15 Minutes Per Day

Resistance Band Workouts for Bad Posture and Back Pain: An Illustrated Resistance Band Exercise Book for Better Posture and Back Pain Relief

DIY Low Back Pain Relief: 9 Ways to Fix Low Back Pain So You Can Feel Like Yourself Again